General Anesthesia as a Multimodal Individualized Clinical Concept

General Anesthesia as a Multimodal Individualized Clinical Concept

Editors

Alexandru Florin Rogobete
Dorel Sandesc

MDPI • Basel • Beijing • Wuhan • Barcelona • Belgrade • Manchester • Tokyo • Cluj • Tianjin

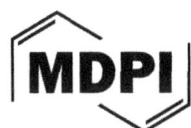

Editors
Alexandru Florin Rogobete
Anaesthesia and Intensive
Care Department, Faculty of
Medicine, "Victor Babes"
University of Medicine
and Pharmacy,
Timisoara, Romania

Dorel Sandesc
Anaesthesia and Intensive
Care Department, Faculty of
Medicine, "Victor Babes"
University of Medicine
and Pharmacy,
Timisoara, Romania

Editorial Office
MDPI
St. Alban-Anlage 66
4052 Basel, Switzerland

This is a reprint of articles from the Special Issue published online in the open access journal *Medicina* (ISSN 1648-9144) (available at: https://www.mdpi.com/journal/medicina/special_issues/general_anesthesia).

For citation purposes, cite each article independently as indicated on the article page online and as indicated below:

LastName, A.A.; LastName, B.B.; LastName, C.C. Article Title. *Journal Name* **Year**, *Volume Number*, Page Range.

ISBN 978-3-0365-5005-3 (Hbk)
ISBN 978-3-0365-5006-0 (PDF)

© 2022 by the authors. Articles in this book are Open Access and distributed under the Creative Commons Attribution (CC BY) license, which allows users to download, copy and build upon published articles, as long as the author and publisher are properly credited, which ensures maximum dissemination and a wider impact of our publications.

The book as a whole is distributed by MDPI under the terms and conditions of the Creative Commons license CC BY-NC-ND.

Contents

Alexandru Florin Rogobete and Dorel Sandesc
General Anesthesia as a Multimodal Individualized
Clinical Concept
Reprinted from: *Medicina* 2022, *58*, 956, doi:10.3390/medicina58070956 1

Ana-Maria Cotae, Mirela Țigliș, Cristian Cobilinschi, Alexandru Emil Băetu, Diana Maria Iacob and Ioana Marina Grințescu
The Impact of Monitoring Depth of Anesthesia and Nociception on Postoperative Cognitive Function in Adult Multiple Trauma Patients
Reprinted from: *Medicina* 2021, *57*, 408, doi:10.3390/medicina57050408 5

Ica Secosan, Delia Virga, Zorin Petrisor Crainiceanu, Lavinia Melania Bratu and Tiberiu Bratu
Infodemia: Another Enemy for Romanian Frontline Healthcare Workers to Fight during the COVID-19 Outbreak
Reprinted from: *Medicina* 2020, *56*, 679, doi:10.3390/medicina56120679 15

Mascha O. Fiedler, Elisabeth Schätzle, Marius Contzen, Christian Gernoth, Christel Weiß, Thomas Walter, Tim Viergutz and Armin Kalenka
Evaluation of Different Positive End-Expiratory Pressures Using Supreme™ Airway Laryngeal Mask during Minor Surgical Procedures in Children
Reprinted from: *Medicina* 2020, *56*, 551, doi:10.3390/medicina56100551 25

Cosmin Balan, Serban-Ion Bubenek-Turconi, Dana Rodica Tomescu and Liana Valeanu
Ultrasound-Guided Regional Anesthesia–Current Strategies for Enhanced Recovery after Cardiac Surgery
Reprinted from: *Medicina* 2021, *57*, 312, doi:10.3390/medicina57040312 35

Alexandru Florin Rogobete, Ovidiu Horea Bedreag, Marius Papurica, Sonia Elena Popovici, Lavinia Melania Bratu, Andreea Rata, Claudiu Rafael Barsac, Andra Maghiar, Dragos Nicolae Garofil, Mihai Negrea, Laura Bostangiu Petcu, Daiana Toma, Corina Maria Dumbuleu, Samir Rimawi and Dorel Sandesc
Multiparametric Monitoring of Hypnosis and Nociception-Antinociception Balance during General Anesthesia—A New Era in Patient Safety Standards and Healthcare Management
Reprinted from: *Medicina* 2021, *57*, 132, doi:10.3390/medicina57020132 51

Mirela Țigliș, Tiberiu Paul Neagu, Andrei Niculae, Ioan Lascăr and Ioana Marina Grințescu
Incidence of Iron Deficiency and the Role of Intravenous Iron Use in Perioperative Periods
Reprinted from: *Medicina* 2020, *56*, 528, doi:10.3390/medicina56100528 69

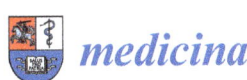

Editorial

General Anesthesia as a Multimodal Individualized Clinical Concept

Alexandru Florin Rogobete [1,2,*] and Dorel Sandesc [1,2]

1. Department of Anaesthesia and Intensive Care, "Victor Babes" University of Medicine and Pharmacy, 300041 Timisoara, Romania; dsandesc@yahoo.com
2. Clinic of Anaesthesia and Intensive Care, Emergency County Hospital "Pius Brinzeu", 325100 Timisoara, Romania
* Correspondence: alexandru.rogobete@umft.ro

Abstract: In the last decades, several new and modern techniques have been developed for the continuous monitoring of vitals for patients undergoing surgery under general anesthesia. These complex methods are meant to come as an adjunct to classical monitoring protocols used in general anesthesia to increase patient safety. The main objectives of multimodal monitoring are avoiding the over- or underdosing of anesthetic drugs, adapting the concentration for the substances in use, reducing post-anesthetic complications, and increasing patient comfort. Recent studies have shown a series of benefits with significant clinical impact such as a reduced incidence of nausea and vomiting, shorter reversal times, a reduction in opioid consumption, shorter hospital stays, and an increase in patient satisfaction.

Keywords: entropy; bispectral index; multimodal monitoring; general anesthesia; electroencefalography

This Special Issue, "General Anesthesia as a Multimodal Individualized Concept", in the *Medicina* journal of MDPI's "Intensive Care/Anesthesiology" section, reports international studies regarding the concept of the personalized monitoring of patients under general anesthesia. Furthermore, it describes modern monitoring techniques for certain anesthesia-specific parameters such as the degree of hypnosis, continuous monitoring of the nociception–antinociception balance, neuromuscular transmission monitoring, and hemodynamic monitoring (heart rate, invasive or non-invasive measurement of blood pressure, peripheral oxygen saturation, temperature). This Special Issue also describes new techniques for monitoring respiratory gases perioperatively by using modern technology such as indirect calorimetry.

Cotae et al., in a randomized prospective study have analyzed the impact that monitoring the degree of hypnosis by using the Entropy technology (E-Entropy Module, GE Healthcare, Helsinki, Finland) and the nociception–antinociception balance through Surgical Pleth Index (SPI Module, GE Healthcare, Helsinki, Finland) can have on postoperative delirium and cognitive dysfunction (POCD) in 107 trauma patients. For the statistical analysis, the authors used two study groups. The first was the target group, in which general anesthesia management was based on multimodal monitoring, and the second group that received classical monitoring in accordance with international guidelines. In the multimodal monitoring group, they studied both Entropy and SPI as constants throughout the general anesthesia. Patient assessment for POCD was based on the Neelon and Champagne (NEECHAM) Confusion Scale. Following this study, they identified statistically significant differences ($p < 0.05$) between the two groups regarding the incidence of POCD, although in the intervention group the overall number was significantly lower [1].

In more detail, Rogobete et al., in their review article "*Multiparametric Monitoring of Hypnosis and Nociception–Antinociception Balance during General Anesthesia—A New Era in Patient Safety Standards and Healthcare Management*", described a series of modern techniques

Citation: Rogobete, A.F.; Sandesc, D. General Anesthesia as a Multimodal Individualized Clinical Concept. *Medicina* 2022, *58*, 956. https://doi.org/10.3390/medicina58070956

Received: 13 July 2022
Accepted: 17 July 2022
Published: 19 July 2022

Publisher's Note: MDPI stays neutral with regard to jurisdictional claims in published maps and institutional affiliations.

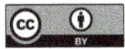

Copyright: © 2022 by the authors. Licensee MDPI, Basel, Switzerland. This article is an open access article distributed under the terms and conditions of the Creative Commons Attribution (CC BY) license (https://creativecommons.org/licenses/by/4.0/).

currently in use in the clinical setting for personalized and individualized general anesthesia monitoring. The group described and summarized information on the most modern monitoring techniques for the degree of hypnosis (Bispectral Index, BIS, Medtronic-Covidien, Dublin, Ireland; Response Entropy/State Entropy, Entropy, GE Healthcare, Hesinki, Findland; Narcotrend index, NCT, Monitor Technik, Germany; and composite auditory evoked potential index, cAAI, AEP Monitor/2, Danmeter A/S, Odense, Denmark). They have also presented recent studies on the topic and have shown the impact of these techniques on hemodynamic stability, incidence of adverse events, anesthetic drug consumption and other quality and safety indicators in medical practice. Furthermore, this review article describes different monitoring techniques for the nociception–antinociception balance and for neuromuscular transmission. The authors also bring to light the impact of general anesthesia on the systemic inflammatory status, oxidative stress, and other biochemical pathways directly or indirectly involved in the clinical outcome of patients undergoing surgery under general anesthesia [2].

Tiglis et al. have published an article—"Incidence of Iron Deficiency and the Role of Intravenous Iron Use in Perioperative Periods"—that shows the importance of the multidisciplinary monitoring of patients undergoing general anesthesia. The research group describes a series of mechanisms and biochemical pathways associated with iron deficit and preoperative anemia, as well as with post-operative low iron levels. Their article presents the impact on clinical prognosis, the direct association between iron deficiency and perioperative need for blood transfusion, incidence of postoperative infection, ICU length of stay, morbidity and mortality, and the economic impact of the medical act [3].

Balan et al., in a review article on ultrasound-based monitoring and diagnosis techniques, underline the importance of ultrasound-guided regional anesthetic techniques on the management of nociception–antinociception balance and the impact of these techniques on opioid consumption, patient satisfaction, and postoperative recovery [4].

Fiedler et al., in an original article, have analyzed a method that is frequently used in ventilatory support for patients under general anesthesia. They carried out an observational trial aiming at evaluating the impact of positive end-expiratory pressure (PEEP) levels on ventilation parameters and gastric air insufflation during laryngeal mask general anesthesia in children. The study only included pediatric patients (n = 67), aged 1 to 11. The authors identified statistically significant differences for ventilatory parameters such as: peak pressure ($p < 0.05$), tidal volume ($p < 0.05$), and dynamic compliance ($p < 0.05$). They reported an increase in all parameters that are directly influenced by the increase of PEEP, except from $etCO_2$, for which they reported a significant increase, and for respiratory rate, for which no differences have been reported. They have also identified a proportional increase in gastric insufflation with increased PEEP. The authors have therefore proven the importance of multimodally monitoring mechanical ventilation during general anesthesia, as well as the fact that modern techniques can reduce side-effects associated with anesthesia [5].

An interesting article, adapted to the crisis that was generated by the COVID-19 pandemic, has been published by Secosan et al., who report on the impact of disinformation regarding SARS-CoV-2 and the impact the pandemic had on the medical personnel. The authors included in their study 100 employees of the Clinic for Anesthesia and Intensive Care in "Pius Brinzeu" Emergency County Hospital in Timisoara, Romania. They all received a questionnaire between March and April 2020 that was meant to evaluate the degree of depression, anxiety, stress, and the incidence of insomnia. The study identified the negative impact that social disinformation had on the stress and anxiety levels of the medical personnel, overlapping with overtime during the crisis, the great number of patients, social and medical drama, the very high number of deaths, and being mentally and physically overworked [6].

In conclusion, this Special Issue presents a number of modern monitoring techniques for all segments of general anesthesia and current clinical practice, presenting updates in the field of monitoring of degree of hypnosis, perioperative pain, neuromuscular transmission, hemodynamic stability, ventilatory support, and the most important biochemical pathways associated with inflammation. Moreover, adapted to the ongoing COVID-19 pandemic, the time of the Special Issue's publication has proven the importance of periodic evaluation of the psychological well-being of medical personnel, as well as the importance of offering psychological support.

Author Contributions: Conceptualization, A.F.R. and D.S.; methodology, A.F.R.; software, A.F.R.; validation, D.S.; formal analysis, A.F.R.; investigation, A.F.R.; resources, A.F.R.; data curation, D.S.; writing—original draft preparation, A.F.R.; writing—review and editing, D.S. and A.F.R.; visualization, D.S.; supervision, D.S.; project administration, A.F.R.; funding acquisition, D.S. All authors have read and agreed to the published version of the manuscript.

Funding: This research received no external funding.

Institutional Review Board Statement: Not applicable.

Informed Consent Statement: Not applicable.

Data Availability Statement: Not applicable.

Acknowledgments: We wish to thank all authors that have contributed to this Special Issue.

Conflicts of Interest: The authors declare no conflict of interest.

References

1. Cotae, A.-M.; Țigliș, M.; Cobilinschi, C.; Băetu, A.; Iacob, D.; Grințescu, I. The Impact of Monitoring Depth of Anesthesia and Nociception on Postoperative Cognitive Function in Adult Multiple Trauma Patients. *Medicina* **2021**, *57*, 408. [CrossRef] [PubMed]
2. Rogobete, A.; Bedreag, O.; Papurica, M.; Popovici, S.; Bratu, L.; Rata, A.; Barsac, C.; Maghiar, A.; Garofil, D.; Negrea, M.; et al. Multiparametric Monitoring of Hypnosis and Nociception-Antinociception Balance during General Anesthesia—A New Era in Patient Safety Standards and Healthcare Management. *Medicina* **2021**, *57*, 132. [CrossRef] [PubMed]
3. Țigliș, M.; Neagu, T.; Niculae, A.; Lascăr, I.; Grințescu, I. Incidence of Iron Deficiency and the Role of Intravenous Iron Use in Perioperative Periods. *Medicina* **2020**, *56*, 528. [CrossRef] [PubMed]
4. Balan, C.; Bubenek-Turconi, S.-I.; Tomescu, D.; Valeanu, L. Ultrasound-Guided Regional Anesthesia–Current Strategies for Enhanced Recovery after Cardiac Surgery. *Medicina* **2021**, *57*, 312. [CrossRef] [PubMed]
5. Fiedler, M.; Schätzle, E.; Contzen, M.; Gernoth, C.; Weiß, C.; Walter, T.; Viergutz, T.; Kalenka, A. Evaluation of Different Positive End-Expiratory Pressures Using Supreme™ Airway Laryngeal Mask during Minor Surgical Procedures in Children. *Medicina* **2020**, *56*, 551. [CrossRef] [PubMed]
6. Secosan, I.; Virga, D.; Crainiceanu, Z.; Bratu, L.; Bratu, T. Infodemia: Another Enemy for Romanian Frontline Healthcare Workers to Fight during the COVID-19 Outbreak. *Medicina* **2020**, *56*, 679. [CrossRef] [PubMed]

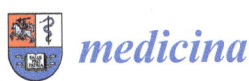

Article

The Impact of Monitoring Depth of Anesthesia and Nociception on Postoperative Cognitive Function in Adult Multiple Trauma Patients

Ana-Maria Cotae [1,2,*], Mirela Țigliș [1,2], Cristian Cobilinschi [1,2], Alexandru Emil Băetu [1,2], Diana Maria Iacob [1,2] and Ioana Marina Grințescu [1,2]

[1] Anaesthesia and Intensive Care Clinic, Clinical Emergency Hospital of Bucharest, 014461 Bucharest, Romania; Mirelatiglis@gmail.com (M.Ț.); cob_rodion@yahoo.com (C.C.); alexandru.baetu@gmail.com (A.E.B.); diana.iacob10@gmail.com (D.M.I.); ioana.grintescu@rospen.ro (I.M.G.)
[2] Department of Anesthesia and Intensive Care, Faculty of Medicine, University of Medicine and Pharmacy Carol Davila, 050474 Bucharest, Romania
* Correspondence: cotae_ana_maria@yahoo.com

Citation: Cotae, A.-M.; Țigliș, M.; Cobilinschi, C.; Băetu, A.E.; Iacob, D.M.; Grințescu, I.M. The Impact of Monitoring Depth of Anesthesia and Nociception on Postoperative Cognitive Function in Adult Multiple Trauma Patients. *Medicina* **2021**, *57*, 408. https://doi.org/10.3390/medicina57050408

Academic Editor: Stefania Mondello

Received: 10 March 2021
Accepted: 20 April 2021
Published: 23 April 2021

Publisher's Note: MDPI stays neutral with regard to jurisdictional claims in published maps and institutional affiliations.

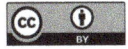

Copyright: © 2021 by the authors. Licensee MDPI, Basel, Switzerland. This article is an open access article distributed under the terms and conditions of the Creative Commons Attribution (CC BY) license (https://creativecommons.org/licenses/by/4.0/).

Abstract: *Background and Objectives*: Patients with traumatic injuries have often been excluded from studies that have attempted to pinpoint modifiable factors to predict the transient disturbance of the cognitive function in the postoperative settings. Anesthetists must be aware of the high risk of developing postoperative delirium and cognitive dysfunction (POCD) in patients undergoing emergency surgery. Monitoring the depth of anesthesia in order to tailor anesthetic delivery may reduce this risk. The primary aim of this study was to improve the prevention strategies for the immediate POCD by assessing anesthetic depth and nociception during emergency surgery. *Material and Methods*: Of 107 trauma ASA physical status II–IV patients aged over 18 years undergoing emergency noncardiac surgery, 95 patients were included in a prospective randomized study. Exclusion criteria were neurotrauma, chronic use of psychoactive substances or alcohol, impaired preoperative cognitive function, pre-existing psychopathological symptoms, or expected surgery time less than 2 h. Entropy and Surgical Pleth Index (SPI) values were constantly recorded for one group during anesthesia. POCD was assessed 24 h, 48 h, and 72 h after surgery using the Neelon and Champagne (NEECHAM) Confusion Scale. *Results*: Although in the intervention group, fewer patients experienced POCD episodes in comparison to the control group, the results were not statistically significant ($p < 0.08$). The study showed a statistically significant inverse correlation between fentanyl and the NEECHAM Confusion Scale at 24 h ($r = -0.32$, $p = 0.0005$) and 48 h ($r = -0.46$, $p = 0.0002$), sevoflurane and the NEECHAM Confusion Scale at 24 h ($r = -0.38$, $p = 0.0014$) and 48 h ($r = -0.52$, $p = 0.0002$), and noradrenaline and POCD events in the first 48 h ($r = -0.46$, $p = 0.0013$ for the first 24 h, respectively, and $r = -0.46$, $p = 0.0002$ for the next 24 h). *Conclusions*: Entropy and SPI monitoring during anesthesia may play an important role in diminishing the risk of developing immediate POCD after emergency surgery.

Keywords: entropy; POCD; general emergency surgery; anesthesia depth

1. Introduction

First described in the mid-20th century, cognitive dysfunction following anesthesia and surgery is a complication that can have a significant impact on patients, leading to unfavorable outcomes [1]. Postoperative cognitive dysfunction (POCD) is described as a decline of the intellectual functions and processes (both basic and higher executive skills) that develops after surgery [2]. Although recognized as a transient decline of cognitive function, POCD can persist for weeks, months, or more. POCD also interferes with patients' psychological status, long-term outcome, mortality, and hospital discharge [3–5].

Postoperative cognitive decline occurs more frequently in the elderly population, with a higher incidence in patients older than 60 years irrespective of the type of anesthesia and surgery. Despite the fact that studies assessing cognitive impairment have been primarily centered on the study of older patients, there is a general agreement that POCD is more likely to occur after major surgery [5,6]. Although this type of cognitive dysfunction is considered multifactorial, it remains difficult to determine whether its occurrence is a result of patient-, surgical-, or anesthesia-related factors [7]. Several risk factors have been suggested to be involved in the pathophysiology of cognitive dysfunction, such as inflammatory cytokines, pain, preoperative impairment in neurocognitive function, metabolic disturbances, duration/type of surgery, hypoxemia, old age, and the use of certain anesthetics (sedation medication or different volatile anesthetic agents) [5–8].

Fortunately, several screening tests are available to establish cognitive disorders. Among these, one stands out for being easily performed without supplemental training. The Neelon and Champagne (NEECHAM) Confusion Scale was developed not only to identify postoperative delirium but also to classify patients as "early to mild confused ", "at risk", or "normal " [9,10]. A score between 0 and 24 points is conclusive for the presence of at least one cognitive impairment. The scale has acceptable sensitivity, specificity, and predictive values when compared to the CAM-ICU [11].

This recent development encourages us to use electroencephalography (EEG) monitoring to assess the depth of anesthesia. Using neuromonitoring during anesthetic delivery can reduce the risk for postoperative cognitive side effects [12]. Among the anesthesia monitors currently approved to assess the depth of anesthesia, the entropy monitor proves to be one of the most reliable. The entropy device is capable of acquiring not only EEG signals but also frontal electromyography data, transforming them into two values: State and response entropy. The entropy device then displays state and response entropy as numerical values, denoting the depth of anesthesia. State entropy and response entropy are given indices between 0–91 and 0–100, respectively, ranging from complete suppression of cortical neuronal activity to an awake-state EEG [13].

As we have already mentioned, another important element in developing POCD is pain. In order to monitor intraoperative nociceptive stimulation and antinociceptive drug effects, different tools have been proposed over the years. Among them, the Surgical Pleth Index (SPI) has received recognition after several studies reported a better outcome in comparison to conventional analgesia. The Surgical Pleth Index module is designed to acquire and process the plethysmograph pulse wave and heartbeat frequency. The parameter has a range of value between 0 and 100. Although there is little to no validation of a specific cut-off value, previous studies have recommended a target value of SPI ≤ 50 [14,15].

The aim of this study was to reduce the incidence of POCD in the first 72 h by assessing anesthetic depth using entropy and nociception through the Surgical Pleth index (SPI) during emergency surgery.

2. Materials and Methods

2.1. Study Design

This prospective randomized study was carried out in the Anaesthesia and Intensive Care Clinic, Clinical Emergency Hospital of Bucharest, between August 2018 and January 2019. All the procedures performed during this study were in accordance with the Declaration of Helsinki.

The study was approved by the Research Ethical Committee of our hospital (registration number 2100/2021), and all the patients provided written informed consent. Patients were considered eligible for the study if they were over 18 years old, undergoing emergency noncardiac surgery expected to last at least 2 h, and American Society of Anesthesiologists (ASA) physical status II, III, or IV. The surgical procedures included abdominal (splenectomy, splenorrhapy, hepatorrhapy, hemicolectomy, phrenoraphy) and orthopedic (femoral osteosynthesis, tibial osteosynthesis, humeral osteosynthesis) surgery. Exclusion criteria were neurotrauma, chronic use of psychoactive substances or alcohol, impaired preoperative cognitive function pre-existing psychopathological symptoms, neurological deficits, or expected surgery time less than 2 h. From the collection data process, we excluded patients intubated prior to the surgical procedure and those who remained intubated at the end of the surgical procedure. The patients were consecutively assigned into 2 study groups. In the first group, anesthesia was provided under standard monitoring (SMG): 5-lead electrocardiogram, noninvasive arterial pressure, pulse oximetry, temperature and end-tidal carbon dioxide concentration. In the second group, apart from standard monitoring, entropy and SPI data were allowed to be included into the management of anesthesia (ESMG).

2.2. Anesthesia

Sedative premedication was prescribed in a dosage of 0.01–0.02 mg/kg midazolam, which was adjusted to the patient's condition. Before induction of anesthesia, entropy electrodes were applied to the patient's forehead as recommended by the manufacturer. Anesthesia was induced using propofol or etomidate (depending on the indications) in combination with fentanyl 2–3 µg/kg, followed by a neuromuscular block to facilitate tracheal intubation with rocuronium 0.6–1 mg/kg. Anesthesia was maintained using a volatile anesthetic (sevoflurane). The anesthesiologists were unrestricted in using conventional regimens of opioid analgesics and neuromuscular blocking agents as required. In order to maintain an anesthetic state in the SM Group, anesthesia was adjusted according to somatic response and hemodynamic events, while in the ESM Group, the anesthesiologists tailored anesthesia to achieve state entropy between 40–60 and an SPI value≤ 50.

2.3. Data Collection, Assesment of Postoperative of POCD, and Delirium

For each patient included in the ESM Group, we recorded the state entropy (SE) and response entropy (RE) in the awakening state, every 15 min after the beginning of surgery and at extubation time. Because negligible differences exist between state and responsive entropy in curarized patients, we decided to acquire only state entropy data. Other data collected included patient characteristics, surgical procedure, anesthetic data, and the intraoperative hemodynamics.

Between the groups, we recorded and compared the incidence of hypotension, bradycardia, tachycardia (variation of more than 20% from preinduction values of mean arterial blood pressure and heart rate). Patients were discharge from the post-anesthesia care unit based on the modified Aldrete score criteria. Postoperative analgesia was guided according to patient demands and consisted of 1 g paracetamol every 6 h, 20 mg nefopam every 12 h, or morphine (0.1 mg/kg) every 8 h, as well as 50–100 mg ketoprofen every12 h in selected cases.

Postoperative cognitive dysfunctions were assessed 24 h, 48 h, and 72 h after surgery using the NEECHAM Confusion Scale. Patients' cognitive status could not be further evaluated because the majority of patients were discharged from ICU after 3 days. Another reason for taking into account only the first 3 postoperative days was other postoperative events that could have interfered with our findings. Screening was performed by trained medical personnel.

2.4. Statistical Analysis

The objective of this study was to demonstrate that the use of entropy and SPI monitoring in assessing anesthetic depth in emergency surgery is associated with a reduction in postoperative cognitive dysfunctions events. GraphPad 8Prism and MedCalc14.1 were used for statistical analysis.

Given the objective of this study, the correlations between the doses of anesthetics used and the NEECHAM score imposed a sufficient sample size to meet this goal. For this calculation, we used the MedCalc program 14.1 (Sampling-Correlation coefficient). We considered it appropriate to use a significance level of 0.05 to avoid the occurrence of a type 1 error (alpha level 2-sided) and 0.1 to avoid the occurrence of a type 2 error (beta) using an input of the correlation coefficient of 0.5 (the hypothesized or anticipated correlation coefficient). At least 29 patients were required for each group and patients were randomized according to the permuted block technique.

The Anderson–Darling test was used to test the data distribution. Data with normal distribution were compared using the student's t-test and presented as mean with SD, and data that did not follow the normal distribution were analyzed using nonparametric tests (Mann–Whitney). Different methods for correlation analyses available from MedCalc14.1 were performed, namely Pearson correlation (r) for Gaussian distribution and Spearman rho for nonparametric data. Nominal data were compared using the chi-square test or Fisher's exact test. A p-value < 0.05 was considered statistically significant.

In order identify how we could avoid postoperative cognitive dysfunction, we developed a logistic regression model that used a NEECHAM score at 24 h higher than 24 (indicating the absence of cognitive dysfunction) as a dependent variable. The logistic regression model included the use of entropy monitoring and doses of fentanyl, sevoflurane, and norepinephrine.

3. Results

Of 107 trauma patients undergoing general emergency noncardiac surgery, 12 patients were excluded from the study after application of the exclusion criteria. The remaining 95 patients were assigned using the permuted block randomization design in a 1:1 ratio to the standard monitoring group (SMG) or to the entropy-SPI standard monitoring group (ESMG). Of these patients, 11 and 10 subjects, respectively, were excluded from data analysis either because they remained intubated at the end of the procedure or because the length of the procedure was less than 2 h (Figure 1).

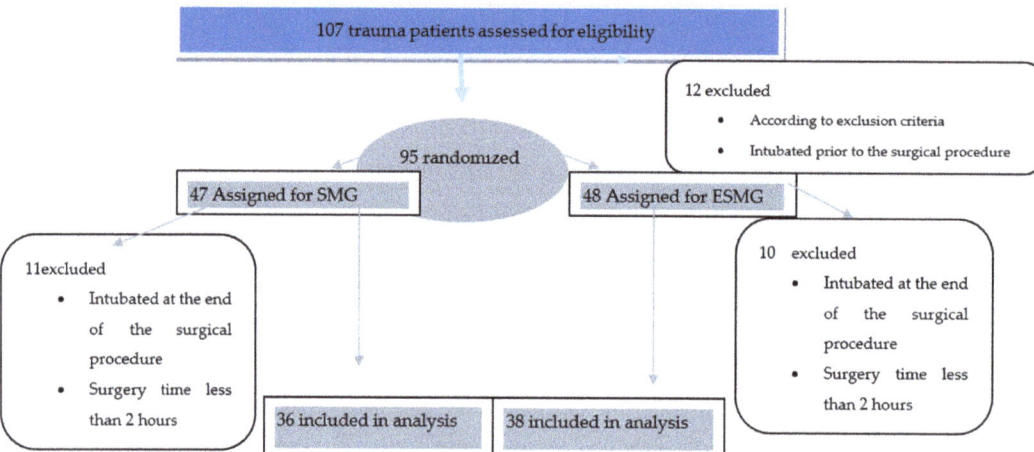

Figure 1. Data collection flowchart.

Patient characteristics were similar in both groups (SMG, ESMG; Table 1), and no significant difference was found in the preoperative data except for the duration of anesthesia. Due to the heterogeneity of trauma patients and the variety of surgical procedures employed, no significant statistical analysis could be performed given the small sample for each group studied. Regarding comorbidities, the most frequently associated pathologies were represented by cardiovascular disease (arterial hypertension, ischemic cardiomyopathy) and obesity.

The total dose of fentanyl administered to patients was lower in the ESM Group than in the SM Group, with a statistically significant difference between the two groups ($p < 0.0001$). Sevoflurane uptake per hour was significantly lower in the study group than in the control group ($p < 0.0001$) (Table 2). Anesthesia length was approximately 17 min shorter in the entropy and SPI monitored group than in the standard monitored group (132.52 vs. 150.05 min, $p = 0.0013$). The shorter anesthesia length in the ESM group might be a cofounding factor with regard to the anesthetic volatile consumption.

Table 1. Patient characteristics.

		SMG (n = 36)	ESMG (n = 38)	p-Value
Gender—Female/male **		15/21	17/21	
ASA Score *, n (%) **	II	12(33.3)	9(23.6)	p = 0.582
	III	17(47.2)	18(47.3)	
	IV	7(19.4)	11(28.9)	

* ASA, American Society of Anesthesiologists. ** Categorical data were expressed as number and percentage.

Table 2. Comparison of entropy and SPI-guided anesthesia in contrast with standard monitoring-guided anesthesia.

Patient Characteristics	Median Group ESMG	Median Group SMG	95%CI for the Median ESMG	95%CI for the Median SMG	Interquartile Range ESMG	Interquartile Range SMG	p-Value
Age	45	44	35.6 to 54.00	36.00 to 57.00	27.5 to 59.5	32.00 to 64.00	0.681
Temperature	36.7	37	36.5 to 36.9	36.7 to 37.1	36.4 to 37.00	36.5 to 37.2	0.024
Fentanyl (μg)	350	500	332.9 to 350.00	450.00 to 500.00	300.00 to 400.00	450.00 to 550.00	<0.001
Sevoflurane(mL/h)	3.2	5.15	3.00 to 3.40	5.00 to 5.3	2.9 to 3.6	4.9 to 5.6	<0.001
Crystalloid (mL)	2500	3250	2500.00 to 3170.52	3000.00 to 4000.00	2500.00 to 3500.00	3000.00 to 4000.00	0.010
Colloid (mL)	1000	1000	500.00 to 1000.00	500.00 to 1000.00	500.00 to 1000.00	500.00 to 1000.00	0.324
Noradrenaline (μg/kg/min)	0.08	1	0.05 to 0.50	0.9 to 1.2	0.05 to 0.5	0.8 to 1.3	<0.001

Data were analyzed using the Mann–Whitney test.

In regard to intraoperative fluid management, fewer fluids were used for the ESM Group, and statistically significant results between the two groups were found only for crystalloid ($p = 0.010$). As for the noradrenaline dosage, the ESM Group received a smaller dose of vasopressor in comparison to the SM Group ($p < 0.0001$) (Table 2).

Hemodynamic events are listed in Table 3. Intraoperative hypotension was encountered more frequently in the control group ($p < 0.0001$). No statistically significant differences were noted between the two groups regarding the incidence of other hemodynamic disturbances.

Table 3. Comparison of entropy and SPI-guided anesthesia in contrast with standard monitoring-guided anesthesia regarding adverse intraoperative hemodynamic events.

	SMG	ESMG	p-Value
At least one intraoperatory episode of			
Tachycardia	10	12	0.61
Bradycardia	10	4	0.13
Hypotension	36	18	0.0001

Nominal data were compared using Fisher's exact test.

Postoperative Delirium and Cognitive Dysfunction

Although fewer patients in the intervention group experienced postoperative cognitive dysfunctions episodes in comparison to the control group, the results were not statistically significant ($p = 0.08$). The study showed a statistically significant inverse correlation between fentanyl and the NEECHAM Confusion Scale at 24 h ($r = -0.32$, $p = 0.0005$) and 48 h ($r = -0.46$, $p = 0.0002$), sevoflurane and the NEECHAM Confusion Scale at 24 h ($r = -0.38$, $p = 0.0014$) and 48 h ($r = -0.52$, $p = 0.0002$), and noradrenaline and POCD events in the first 48 h ($r = -0.46$, $p = 0.0013$ for the first 24 h respectively, and $r = -0.46$, $p = 0.0002$

for the next 24 h) (Figure 2). There was no statistically significant correlation between fentanyl, sevoflurane, or noradrenaline and POCD at 72 h (Figure 2).

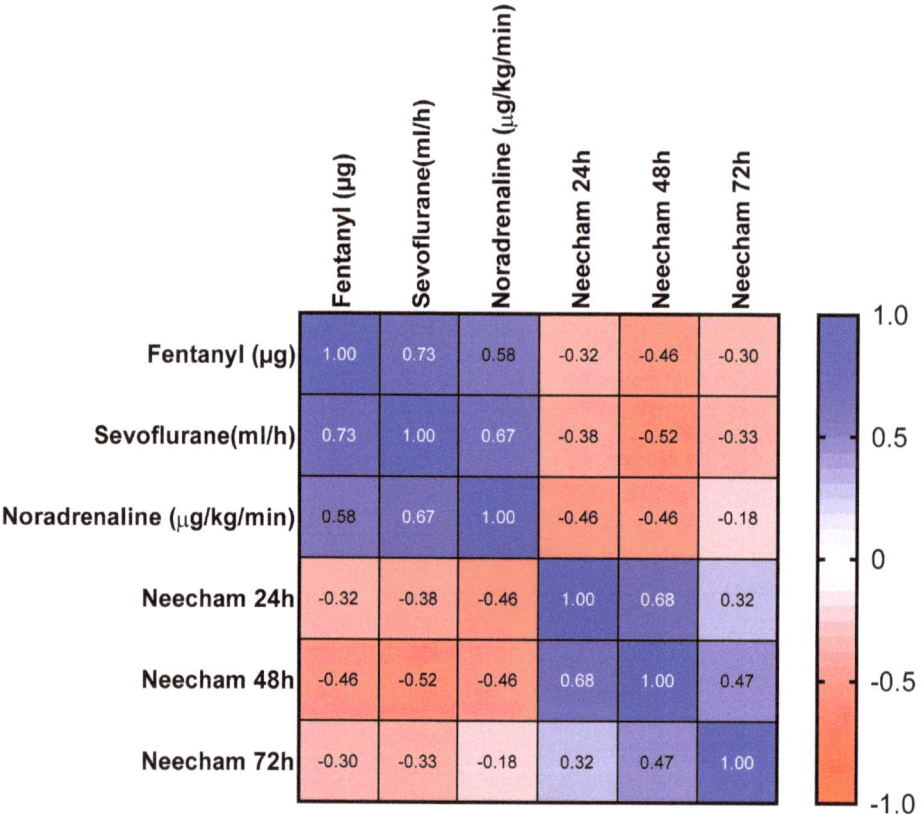

Figure 2. Correlation matrix. The table above shows correlations coefficients between the following variables: Fentanyl (μg), sevoflurane (mL/h), noradrenaline (μg/kg/min) and NEECHAM score at 24 h, 48 h, and 72 h. The colorencodes the sign of correlation between each 2 variables: Blue for positive r values and red for negative r values.

In order to identify how we couldavoid postoperative cognitive dysfunction, we developed a logistic regression model that used a NEECHAM score higher than 24 points (indicating absence of cognitive dysfunction) at 24 h as a dependent variable. A four-predictor logistic model was fitted to the data to test the research hypothesis regarding the relationship between the use of entropy and the doses of anesthetic drugs and vasopressor with the advent of postoperative cognitive dysfunctions.

The logistic regression hadan overall model fit described by a nullmodel-2 Log Likelihood of 74.150 and a full model-2 Log Likelihood of 65.311, with a chi-squared value of 8.840 ($p = 0.06$). The goodness of fit of this regression model was calculated with Cox&Snell ($R^2 = 0.19$). According to the model, the log of the odds of a patient to develop POCD was negatively related to the dose of fentanyl, sevoflurane, or noradrenaline and positively related toentropy and SPI monitoring (Table 4).

Table 4. Logistic regression analysis of 74 patients for POCD appearance.

Coefficient and Standard Errors				
Variable	Coefficient	Std.Error	Wald	P
ESMG = 1	4.1	1.8	5.2	0.022
Fentanyl µg	0.006	0.004	1.7	0.182
Noradrenaline µg/kg/min	0.4	0.7	0.3	0.541
Sevoflurane mL/h	0.7	0.7	1.08	0.296
Constant	−7.4	4.3	2.8	0.090

Odds Ratios and 95% Confidence Intervals		
Variable	Odds Ratio	95%CI
ESMG = 1	66.1	1.8 to 2423.3
Fentanyl µg	1.006	0.9 to 1.01
Noradrenaline µg/kg/min	1.5	0.3 to 7.03
Sevoflurane mL/h	2.1	0.5 to 9.3

4. Discussion

The main finding of this study was that entropy and Surgical Pleth Index-guided anesthesia versus standard monitoring may reduce the incidence of postoperative cognitive dysfunction in the first 72 h for patients undergoing general emergency noncardiac surgery. Also, entropy and SPI may offer a protective role in developing postoperative cognitive dysfunctions. The reported incidence varies greatly in the literature [16,17], especially because neuromonitoring anesthesia has been studied less during emergency noncardiac surgery in comparison to elective surgery.

In our research, we found a substantial reduction in anesthesia duration in the entropy and Surgical PlethIndexmonitored group than in the standard monitored group (132.52 vs. 150.05 min, $p = 0.0013$). The shorter anesthesia length in the ESM Group might be a confounding factor with regard to the anesthetic volatile consumption. In our study, we observed significantly lower sevoflurane doses in the ESM Group. Previous studies demonstrated that neuromonitoring may lead to a less 'roller-coaster'-like anesthesia [18] and less fluctuation from a defined target than the clinical estimation of anesthetic depth only [19]. Hor et al. conducted a randomized controlled trial in order to assess sevoflurane uptake in patients undergoing major surgery andfounda significant reduction in sevoflurane uptake with the use of entropy, in addition to a faster extubation [20]. Fedorow et al. highlighted that using neuromonitoring in order totitrateanesthetic agents may avoid an unnecessary increase in anesthesialevels and possible neurotoxic effects, especially in high-risk patients [21]. Our data suggest that anesthetic agents may represent a risk factor for developing POCD in the first 48 h. This finding is consistent with previouslypublished studies. According to Micha et al., sevoflurane has a negative influence on short-termcognition [22].

Another pharmacological factor, fentanyl, can be considered a causal factor for the presence of POCD, and we have identified significant dose reduction in the entropy-SPI monitored group in comparison to the standard monitored group. In our study, we identified that fentanyl may represent a risk factor for developing POCD in the first 48 h, but the results cannot be extended topatients who develop POCD in the next 24 h. Although the incidence of cognitive disorders is highly dependent on the type of surgery and general anesthesia management [23,24], opioid treatment remains very influential in POCD occurrence [25].

Emergency surgery is usually closely related to hemodynamic instability. Thus, another favorable trend for the entropy-SPI studied group is represented by fewer hypotensive eventsin the intervention group and by the significantly decreased demand for vasopressor. Intraoperative hypotension was encountered more frequently in the control group ($p < 0.0001$). It is well known that, in addition to uncontrolled anesthetic exposure, another important factor that may increase the risk of developing POCD is represented by blood pressure fluctuation [26,27]. As Wu et al. investigated in a randomized controlled trial, this may be related to sevoflurane consumption [28]. However, we must keep in mind that, in trauma settings, other important factors may contribute to hemodynamic alteration (type of injury, intravascular volemic status, volemic resuscitation, response to tissue injury, tissue perfusion, etc.) [29]. Our findings highlight that noradrenaline may contribute to cognitive impairment in the first 48 h after surgery. Although vasopressors are a cornerstone for treating refractory hypovolemic shock, they may also exhibit negative side effects with harmful repercussion on cerebral perfusion [30,31].

In our study, the majority of patients experienced the following comorbidities: Cardiovascular disease (arterial hypertension, ischemic cardiomyopathy) and obesity. Current data do not support the hypothesis that these comorbidities are potential cofounders for developing postoperative cognitive dysfunctions [32,33].

5. Limits

Although in the intervention group, fewer patients experienced postoperative cognitive dysfunctions episodes in comparison to the control group, the results were not statistically significant ($p < 0.08$). We consider that one of the main drawbacks of the study was the inability to control all of the risk factors that contribute to the development cognitive disorders.

Another study limitation is the consequence of not being to further evaluate postoperative cognitive disorders after 72 h because the majority of patients were discharged from ICU. We also considered that, after 72 h, other factors may interfere with cognitive function and mislead POCD screening.

Due to the fact that neuromonitoring anesthesia and nociception have been studied less frequently during emergency noncardiac surgery in comparison to elective surgery, the available papers do not allow us to entirely compare the magnitude of our findings with the previous published data.

The present research included a small number of patients in each group. In order to establish future relevant knowledge for improving patients' cognitive outcome, we con-sider it imperative to recruit a higher number of patients.

6. Conclusions

The present study was designed to reflect routine clinical practice in emergency settings. It is difficult to isolate one perioperative risk factor for POCD in studies even when excluding individual factors. Despite the extensive research conducted in recent years on the subject, the causes and pathophysiological mechanisms responsible for postoperative cognitive decline remain unclear. Entropy and SPI monitoring during anesthesia may play an important role in diminishing the risk of developing immediate postoperative cognitive dysfunctions after emergency surgery. Also, sevoflurane, fentanyl, and noradrenaline may be closely associated with POCD occurrence in the first 48 h. In order to confirm our hypothesis, we considered that our study required a higher number of patients to be enrolled. Building upon the data found in our research, we suggest monitoring intraoperative anesthetic depth using entropy and nociception through the SurgicalPlethIndex (SPI) in patients with pre-existing cognitive impairment in order to investigate postoperative cognitive dysfunction in future research.

Author Contributions: Conceptualization, A.-M.C., C.C., M.Ț. and I.M.G.; Data curation, A.-M.C., C.C., M.Ț., A.E.B. and D.M.I.; Formal analysis, A.E.B.; Investigation, A.-M.C., C.C., M.Ț., A.E.B. and D.M.I.; Methodology, A.-M.C., C.C., M.Ț. and I.M.G.; Project administration, A.-M.C. and I.M.G.; Resources, C.C. and I.M.G.; Software, A.E.B. and D.M.I.; Supervision, D.M.I. and I.M.G.; Validation, A.-M.C., C.C., M.Ț. and A.E.B.; Visualization, I.M.G.; Writing—original draft, A.-M.C., C.C., M.Ț., A.E.B., D.M.I. and I.M.G. All authors have read and agreed to the published version of the manuscript.

Funding: This research received no external funding.

Institutional Review Board Statement: This prospective randomized study was carried out in the Anaesthesia and Intensive Care Clinic, Clinical Emergency Hospital of Bucharest, between August

2018 and January 2019. All the procedures performed during this study were in accordance with the Dec-laration of Helsinki. The study was approved by the Research Ethical Committee of our hospital (registration number 2100/2021).

Informed Consent Statement: All the patients provided written informed consent.

Data Availability Statement: No data were reported.

Conflicts of Interest: The authors declare no conflict of interest.

References

1. Bedford, P.D. Adverse cerebral effects of anaesthesia on old people. *Lancet* **1955**, *266*, 259–263. [CrossRef]
2. Ramaiah, R. What's new in emergencies, trauma and shock? Anesthesia, surgery and postoperative cognition. *J. Emergencies Trauma Shock* **2011**, *4*, 1–2. [CrossRef]
3. Kotekar, N.; Shenkar, A.; Nagaraj, R. Postoperative cognitive dysfunction—Current preventive strategies. *Clin. Interv. Aging* **2018**, *13*, 2267–2273. [CrossRef]
4. Rundshagen, I. Postoperative cognitive dysfunction. *Dtsch. Arztebl. Int.* **2014**, *111*, 119–125. [CrossRef] [PubMed]
5. Newman, S.D.; Stygall, J.; Hirani, S.; Shaefi, S.; Maze, M. Postoperative cognitive dysfunction after noncardiac surgery: A systematic review. *Anesthesiology* **2007**, *106*, 572–590. [CrossRef]
6. Monk, T.G.; Weldon, B.C.; Garvan, C.W.; Dede, D.E.; Van Der Aa, M.T.; Heilman, K.M.; Gravenstein, J.S. Predictors of cognitive dysfunction after major noncardiac surgery. *Anesthesiology* **2008**, *108*, 18–30. [CrossRef]
7. Culley, D.J.; Monk, T.G.; Cosby, G. *Post-Operative Central Nervous System Dysfunction, Geriatric Anaesthesiology*, 2nd ed.; Springer: New York, NY, USA, 2018; Volume 9, pp. 123–136.
8. Steinmetz, J.; Christensen, K.B.; Lund, T.; Lohse, N.; Rasmussen, L.S.; ISPOCD Group. Long-term consequences of postoperative cognitive dysfunction. *Anesthesiology* **2009**, *110*, 548–555. [CrossRef] [PubMed]
9. Neelon, V.J.; Champagne, M.T.; Carlson, J.R.; Funk, S.G. The NEECHAM Confusion Scale: Construction, validation, and clinical testing. *Nurs. Res.* **1996**, *45*, 324–330. [CrossRef] [PubMed]
10. Polderman, K.H. Screening methods for delirium: Don't get confused! *Intensive Care Med.* **2007**, *33*, 3–5. [CrossRef]
11. Van Rompaey, B.; Schuurmans, M.J.; Shortridge-Baggett, L.M.; Truijen, S.; Elseviers, M.; Bossaert, L. A comparison of the CAM-ICU and the NEECHAM Confusion Scale in intensive care delirium assessment: An observational study in non-intubated patients. *Crit Care* **2008**, *12*, R16. [CrossRef] [PubMed]
12. Green, D.; Ballard, C.; Kunst, G. Depth of anaesthesiaoptimisation and postoperative cognitive dysfunction. *BJA Br. J.* **2015**, *114*, 343–344. [CrossRef] [PubMed]
13. Viertio-Oja, H.; Maja, V.; Sarkela, M.; Talja, P.; Tenkanen, N.; Tolvanen-Laakso, H.; Paloheimo, M.; Vakkuri, A.; Yli-Hankala, A. Description of the Entropy (TM) algorithm as applied in the Datex-Ohmeda S/5 (TM) Entropy Module. *Acta Anaesthesiol. Scand.* **2004**, *48*, 154–161. [CrossRef] [PubMed]
14. Won, Y.J.; Lim, B.G.; Kim, Y.S.; Lee, M.; Kim, H. Usefulness of surgical pleth index-guided analgesia during general anesthesia: A systematic review and meta-analysis of randomized controlled trials. *J. Int. Med. Res.* **2018**, *46*, 4386–4398. [CrossRef]
15. Bonhomme, V.; Uutela, K.; Hans, G.; Maquoi, I.; Born, J.D.; Brichant, J.F.; Lamy, M.; Hans, P. Comparison of the surgical Pleth Index™ with haemodynamic variables to assess nociception-anti-nociception balance during general anaesthesia. *Br. J. Anaesth.* **2011**, *106*, 101–111. [CrossRef]
16. Ancelin, M.L.; de Roquefeuil, G.; Ledésert, B.; Bonnel, F.; Cheminal, J.C.; Ritchie, K. Exposure to anaesthetic agents, cognitive functioning and depressive symptomatology in the elderly. *Br. J. Psychiatry* **2001**, *178*, 360–366. [CrossRef]
17. Chan, M.T.V.; Cheng, B.C.P.; Lee, T.M.C.; Gin, T.; Coda Trial Group. BIS-guided anesthesia decreases postoperative delirium and cognitive decline. *J. Neurosurg. Anesthesiol.* **2013**, *25*, 33–42. [CrossRef]
18. Chen, X.; Thee, C.; Gruenewald, M.; Wnent, J.; Illies, C.; Hoecker, J.; Hanss, R.; Steinfath, M.; Bein, B. Comparison of surgical stress index-guided analgesia with standard clinical practice during routine general anesthesia: A pilot study. *Anesthesiology* **2010**, *112*, 1175–1183. [CrossRef] [PubMed]
19. Rundshagen, I.; Hardt, T.; Cortina, K.; Pragst, F.; Fritzsche, T.; Spies, C. Narcotrend-assisted propofol/remifentanil anaesthesia vs clinical practice: Does it make a difference? *Br. J. Anaesth.* **2007**, *99*, 686–693. [CrossRef]
20. Hor, T.; Linden, P.; Hert, S.; Mélot, C.; Bidgoli, J. Impact of entropy monitoring on volatile anesthetic uptake. *Anesthesiology* **2013**, *118*, 868–873. [CrossRef]
21. Fedorow, C.; Grocott, H.P. Cerebral monitoring to optimize outcomes after cardiac surgery. *Curr. Opin. Anaesthesiol.* **2010**, *23*, 89–94. [CrossRef]
22. Micha, G.; Tzimas, P.; Zalonis, I.; Kotsis, K.; Papdopoulos, G.; Arnaoutoglou, E. Propofol vs Sevoflurane anaesthesia on postoperative cognitive dysfunction in the elderly. A randomized controlled trial. *Acta Anaesthesiol. Belg.* **2016**, *67*, 129–137.
23. Jiahai, M.; Xueyan, W.; Yonggang, X.; Jianhong, Y.; Qunhui, H.; Zhi, L.; Juan, D.; Xiuliang, J. Spectral entropy monitoring reduces anesthetic dosage for patients undergoing off-pump coronary artery bypass graft surgery. *J. Cardiothorac. Vasc. Anesth.* **2012**, *26*, 818–821. [CrossRef] [PubMed]

24. Gruenewald, M.; Zhou, J.; Schloemerkemper, N.; Meybohm, P.; Weiler, N.; Tonner, P.H.; Scholz, J.; Bein, B. M-Entropy guidance vs standard practice during propofol-remifentanil anaesthesia: A randomised controlled trial. *Anaesthesia* **2007**, *62*, 1224–1229. [CrossRef]
25. MacKenzie, K.K.; Britt-Spells, A.M.; Sands, L.P.; Leung, J.M. Processed Electroencephalogram Monitoring and Postoperative Delirium: A Systematic Review and Meta-analysis. *Anesthesiology* **2018**, *129*, 417–427. [CrossRef] [PubMed]
26. Hirsch, J.; DePalma, G.; Tsai, T.T.; Sands, L.P.; Leung, J.M. Impact of intraoperative hypotension and blood pressure fluctuations on early postoperative delirium after non-cardiac surgery. *Br. J. Anaesth.* **2015**, *115*, 418–426. [CrossRef] [PubMed]
27. Selnes, O.A.; McKhann, G.M. Neurocognitive complications after coronary artery bypass surgery. *Ann. Neurol.* **2005**, *57*, 615–621. [CrossRef] [PubMed]
28. Wu, S.C.; Wang, P.C.; Liao, W.T.; Shih, T.H.; Chang, K.A.; Lin, K.C.; Chou, A.K. Use of spectral entropy monitoring in reducing the quantity of sevoflurane as sole inhalational anesthetic and in decreasing the need for antihypertensive drugs in total knee replacement surgery. *Acta Anaesthesiol. Taiwanica.* **2008**, *46*, 106–111. [CrossRef]
29. Ansaloni, L.; Catena, F.; Chattat, R.; Fortuna, D.; Franceschi, C.; Mascitti, P.; Melotti, R.M. Risk factors and incidence of postoperative delirium in elderly patients after elective and emergency surgery. *Br. J. Surg.* **2010**, *97*, 273–280. [CrossRef] [PubMed]
30. Brassard, P.; Seifert, T.; Secher, N.H. Is cerebral oxygenation negatively affected by infusion of norepinephrine in healthy subjects? *Br. J. Anaesth.* **2009**, *102*, 800–805. [CrossRef]
31. Müller, S.; How, O.-J.; Hermansen, S.E.; Stenberg, T.A.; Sager, G.; Myrmel, T. Vasopressin impairs brain, heart and kidney perfusion: An experimental study in pigs after transient myocardial ischemia. *Crit Care* **2008**, *12*, R20. [CrossRef]
32. Feinkohl, I.; Winterer, G.; Pischon, T. Hypertension and Risk of Post-Operative Cognitive Dysfunction (POCD): A Systematic Review and Meta-Analysis. *Clin. Pract. Epidemiol. Ment. Health* **2017**, *13*, 27–42. [CrossRef] [PubMed]
33. Feinkohl, I.; Winterer, G.; Pischon, T. Obesity and post-operative cognitive dysfunction: A systematic review and meta-analysis. *Diabetes Metab. Res. Rev.* **2016**, *32*, 643–651. [CrossRef] [PubMed]

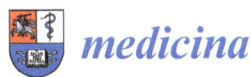

Article

Infodemia: Another Enemy for Romanian Frontline Healthcare Workers to Fight during the COVID-19 Outbreak

Ica Secosan [1], Delia Virga [2,*], Zorin Petrisor Crainiceanu [1], Lavinia Melania Bratu [1] and Tiberiu Bratu [1]

1. Faculty of Medicine, "Victor Babes" University of Medicine and Pharmacy, 300041 Timisoara, Romania; secosan.ica@umft.ro (I.S.); zcrainiceanu@gmail.com (Z.P.C.); lavinia.melania.bratu@gmail.com (L.M.B.); office@brol.ro (T.B.)
2. Department of Psychology, West University of Timisoara, 325100 Timisoara, Romania
* Correspondence: delia.virga@e-uvt.ro

Received: 2 November 2020; Accepted: 7 December 2020; Published: 9 December 2020

Abstract: *Background and Objectives:* The population has been overwhelmed with false information related to the Coronavirus disease (COVID-19) crisis, spreading rapidly through social media and other channels. We aimed to investigate if frontline healthcare workers affected by infodemia show different psychological consequences than frontline clinicians who do not declare to be affected by false news related to the COVID-19 pandemic. *Materials and Methods:* One hundred twenty-six frontline healthcare workers from the Intensive Care Unit (ICU) and Emergency Departments in Romania completed a survey to assess stress, depression, anxiety, and sleep disorders, between March and April 2020. We split the sample of frontline healthcare workers into two groups based on the self-evaluated criteria: if they were or were not affected by infodemia in their activity. *Results:* Considering limitations such as the cross-sectional design, the lack of causality relationship, and the sample size, the results show that, the frontline medical workers who declared to be affected by false news were significantly more stressed, felt more anxiety, and suffered more from insomnia than healthcare workers who are not affected by false information related to pandemic time. *Conclusions:* The infodemia has significant psychological consequences such as stress, anxiety, and insomnia on already overwhelmed doctors and nurses in the outbreak of the COVID-19 crisis. These findings suggest that medical misinformation's psychological implications must be considered when different interventions regarding frontline healthcare workers during the COVID-19 pandemic are implemented.

Keywords: false news; COVID-19; frontline clinicians; misinformation; stress; mental health; anxiety; insomnia

1. Introduction

As the coronavirus has spread across the world, so too the misinformation about it was exploded. The first cases of COVID-19 in Romania emerged in March 2020. By October, there were 222,559 infected, 6681 deaths, and 27,280 people in isolation. As the virus spreads across the country, the need for information has become a daily preoccupation for many people. Romanian Government created a Strategic Communication Group, which is qualified to communicate information about COVID-19 cases, treatment, and other social and medical implications. Nevertheless, most people rely on social media and look for information on social media platforms instead of using official communication channels.

Before the outbreak of COVID-19, people in many countries already relied on social media to gather information and news. Since the outbreak at the end of 2019, people worldwide return to social media, online press, or television to obtain as much information as they can [1]. A previous study showed that social media played an essential role in the COVID-19 outbreak in most countries. This role is highlighted in three areas: accurate information about the novel coronavirus was published on social media all over the world; fake news and misinformation about the outbreak were published daily on the internet, and social media has played an important role in creating and disseminating fear and panic about the outbreak worldwide [2].

According to *The New York Times*, medical misinformation about the novel coronavirus has been spread by ideologues who do not believe in modern medicine and scientifically proven treatments, like vaccines, and by profiteers who found an opportunity to promote cures or other wellness products [3]. Furthermore, specialists talk about an infodemic of misinformation. Infodemic is a blend of "information" and "epidemic", that refers to disseminating information, both accurate and inaccurate, about an important subject, as a disease. Once the information is spread, it becomes challenging to learn essential information about the topic. The word infodemic was first used in 2003 and has seen renewed usage since the outbreak of the COVID-19 crisis [4].

According to the World Health Organization (WHO), the COVID-19 related infodemic is just as dangerous as the virus itself. Misinformation, disinformation, and rumors during a health emergency, false preventive measures, fake remedies, conspiracy theories, and other incorrect information may have consequences beyond public health [5]. Since the COVID-19 outbreak in Romania, false information is spreading faster than the virus itself. The Romanian government and medical public health experts repeatedly warned against the negative consequences of some of the most viral false medical information, such as: the virus does not exist, the pharmaceutical giants invented the pandemic, vitamin C treats coronavirus, 5G is the source of the virus, people are paid to declare that they are infected with the novel coronavirus, and other misinformation. Infodemics can hamper a significant public health response and create confusion and distrust among people [6]. A past study illustrated the potential of using social media to conduct "infodemiology" studies for public health. Influenza A virus subtype H1N1 (H1N1) pandemic-related tweets on Twitter were used to disseminate official information from credible sources to the public and a source of opinions and experiences. The researchers proved the correlation between the prevalence of misinformation, terminology use, fear, and panic spread publicly, and the correlation between case incidence and public preoccupation [7]. During a pandemic, healthcare professionals should cooperate with the mass media and help identify the inaccurate, and misleading headlines that agitate members of the public, cause fear, impinge on public communication, and diminish countermeasures for the outbreak [8]. In a pandemic, people's emotional reactions are likely to be very complicated and extensive, such as extreme fear and uncertainty. Furthermore, anxiety and distorted perceptions of risk will lead to negative social behaviors [9].

To our knowledge, little evidence is available on the impact of false information during the outbreak of the novel coronavirus (SARS COV2) on the general population and healthcare workers. Misinformation and fake health news in social media may constitute a potential threat to public health. Patients are more likely to mistrust the medical information and disrespect the preventive measures and the medical experts' policies. Furthermore, considering previous studies on misinformation's impact on mental health, false news may negatively impact medical staff. During the COVID-19 outbreak, faced with unprecedented challenges, doctors and nurses must manage levels of stress and trauma similar to ones usually experienced in war zones [10]. We already know from previous studies that during the outbreak of COVID-19, healthcare workers screened positive for moderate to severe levels of depression, anxiety, and stress [11].

Considering these factors, the sample of frontline healthcare workers were split into two groups based on the self-evaluated criteria: if they were or were not affected by infodemia in their activity, we aimed to investigate whether frontline healthcare workers who declared to be affected by false news show different levels of stress, anxiety, depression, and insomnia than frontline clinicians who do not consider themselves to be affected by infodemia related to the COVID-19 pandemic.

In summary, we hypothesize that frontline workers who were declared to be affected by false news are more likely to experience stress, anxiety, depression, and insomnia than healthcare workers who were not affected by fake news in their professional activity.

Hypothesis 1 (H1). *Frontline healthcare workers who are declared to be affected by infodemia have a higher stress level than frontline clinicians who do not claim to be affected by false news.*

Hypothesis 2 (H2). *Frontline medical clinicians affected by infodemia presented a higher level of anxiety than healthcare workers who are not affected by false information.*

Hypothesis 3 (H3). *Frontline medical professionals who are declared to be affected by infodemia experienced a higher level of depression than their colleagues who are not affected by misinformation.*

Hypothesis 4 (H4). *Frontline healthcare workers who claim to be affected by infodemia have a higher incidence of insomnia than frontline professionals who are not affected by false news.*

2. Procedure and Participants

We have surveyed frontline healthcare workers, emergency doctors, ICU doctors, and medical nurses from two Hospital Departments (Emergency and ICU) in Romania, namely the County Emergency Clinical Hospital Pius Brinzeu, Timisoara. The present study is a cross-sectional one; all data were collected from March to April 2020. The study was conducted following the Declaration of Helsinki and approved by the Ethics Committee of the County Emergency Clinical Hospital, No. 170/05.08.2019, as part of ongoing research considering the burnout syndrome and psychological implications healthcare profession. All gathered information was confidential; the participation was entirely voluntary, and written informed consent was obtained from all the participants.

The inclusion criteria concerned the categories of personnel who directly contact patients during the COVID-19 outbreak through the performed medical act, respectively, primary doctors, specialists, residents (trainees), ICU, and emergency medicine nurses. All data were collected online via a link sent by email. A total of 126 health professionals took part in the survey: 32 nurses and 94 physicians were questioned. Sociodemographic data were collected on gender (male or female), marital status (single, married, divorced, widowed), parental status (children; yes or no), profession (physician or nurse), technical title (trainee, specialist, primary or other), and specialty (ICU or emergency medicine specialist).

The Plan of measures for hospitals' preparation in the COVID-19 pandemic, stated by the Romanian Ministry of Health Order number 533/03.29.2020, disposed of by the end of March 2020, that The County Emergency Hospital Pius Brinzeu Timisoara, Romania will take over the critical cases of patients infected with the novel coronavirus. The usual hospital activity was decreased by 80% regarding chronic cases to increase the hospital's resources in treating COVID-19 patients [12]. By May 2020, 19,133 COVID-19 patients in Romania, 98,403 people in isolation, and 2993 people in official quarantine. Although Timis County had, by the end of May, 505 confirmed cases since the outbreak of the novel coronavirus crisis in Romania in early March, the increase in demand and changes to supply, redeployment of staff, extended work tasks the reorganization of hospital facilities, increase in donning and doffing personal protective equipment (PPE) and implementing new guidelines and protocols, caused tremendous psychological pressure for the frontline healthcare workers [13].

3. Materials and Methods

The Depression, Anxiety, and Stress Scale (DASS 21) is a reliable and suitable questionnaire to assess symptoms of common mental health problems, such as depression, anxiety, and stress. This scale's essential function is to evaluate the severity of the core symptoms of depression, anxiety, and stress; thus, it supports our research questions. The DASS 21, as a self-report questionnaire consisting of 21 items, has 7 items per subscale: depression (e.g., "I couldn't seem to experience any positive feeling at all."—the Cronbach's alpha for this scale was $\alpha = 0.88$), anxiety (e.g., "I was worried about situations in which I might panic and make a fool of myself."—the Cronbach's alpha for this scale was $\alpha = 0.88$), and stress (e.g., "I felt that I was rather touchy."—the Cronbach's alpha for this scale was $\alpha = 0.91$). Depression refers to depressed mood, dysphoria, loss of interest and pleasure, anhedonia, and increased fatigue; anxiety refers to agitation, impatience, trouble concentrating, irritability, restlessness, difficulty relaxing, and difficulty falling asleep, while the third factor labeled stress refers to emotional or physical tension. The items are evaluated on a Likert scale, from 0 (did not apply to me at all) to 3 (applied to me very much) [14].

The Insomnia Severity Index (ISI) is a valid a reliable instrument to assess cases of insomnia in the population, with a good psychometric properties The ISI is composed of seven items (e.g., "How worried/distressed are you about your current sleep problem?"), rated on a five-point Likert scale ('0'—not at all, '4'—extremely), and the time interval is 'in the last two weeks'. Cronbach's alpha for this scale was 0.91 [15].

Before the study's beginning, we organized a focus group with respondents from the ICU and Emergency Department, doctors, and nurses. We disseminated two directions and created custom-made questions following these recommendations. The frontline healthcare workers suffered from the false news impact in two ways: they are exposed to medical misinformation and need to make an effort to discern the actual news, and on the other hand, the doctor-patient relationship is affected, patients been themselves exposed to false news and having troubles trusting the medical system and the healthcare specialists. Therefore, specific questions related to fake news influence on the frontline medical staff were created, such as: "Are you affected by fake news in the course of your professional activity?", "In what way fake news affects you?", "What is the word that best describes the media position (print, audiovisual, online press) regarding medical staff during the outbreak of COVID-19?".

We have used the Statistical Package for Social Science (SPSS) v. 21 program (IBM Corp., Armonk, NY, USA). to test our hypothesis. The significance level adopted was $p \leq 0.05$. Independent Student t-tests between two independent groups for all the variables were calculated.

4. Results

Demographic data were self-reported by the participants, as follows: gender (35.7% male and 64.3% female), marital status (42.8% single, 52.3% married, and 4.7% divorced), children (55.5% yes, 44.4% no), profession (74.6% physician, 25.3% nurse), staff category-doctors (45.2% trainee, 15% specialist, 16.6% primary, 23% other), and specialty (36.5% ICU and 63.4% EM) (Table 1), During the study period, the County Emergency Clinical Hospital Pius Brînzeu, Timisoara, was actively involved in the care of COVID-19 patients.

We split the sample of frontline healthcare workers into two groups based on the *criteria*: if they were or were not affected by fake news in their professional activity. We compared these groups concerning stress, depression, anxiety, and also insomnia (Table 2).

The frontline medical workers who were declared to be affected by false news ($N_1 = 43$) were significantly more stressed ($t = 3.04$, $p < 0.001$) than healthcare workers who are not affected by misinformation related to pandemic time ($N_2 = 83$), and this result offers support for Hypothesis 1. The healthcare workers who are affected by infodemia ($N_1 = 43$) feel more anxiety ($t = 1.91$, $p < 0.05$) than healthcare workers who are not affected by false news ($N_2 = 83$), supporting Hypothesis 2. Regarding Hypothesis 3, we found no difference in the level of depression between the frontline clinicians who are declared to be affected by false news ($N_1 = 43$) and their colleagues who claim not to be affected by infodemia related to pandemic times ($t = 1.54$, $p < 0.12$). Consistent with Hypothesis 4, the frontline workers who are affected by misinformation suffer more from insomnia ($t = 1.89$, $p < 0.05$) than healthcare workers who are not affected by the infodemia related to pandemic time ($N_2 = 83$).

Table 1. Demographic and professional characteristics of frontline healthcare workers.

Variables	Categories	Frequency	Percentage
Gender	Male	45	35.7
	Female	81	64.3
	Total	126	100
Marital status	Single	54	42.8
	Married	66	52.3
	Divorced	6	4.7
	Widower	0	0
	Total	126	100
Children	Yes	70	55.5
	No	56	44.4
	Total	126	100
Profession	Physician	94	74.6
	Nurse	32	25.3
	Total	126	100
Staff category-doctors	Trainee	57	45.2
	Specialist	19	15
	Primary	21	16.6
	Other	29	23
	Total	126	100
Specialty	ICU	46	36.5
	EM	80	63.4
	Total	126	100

Table 2. Statistical indicators of differences.

	Variables	N	Mean	t-Test	p
Stress	Affected by fake news	43	7.23	3.04	0.00
	Not affected by fake news	83	4.71		
Depression	Affected by fake news	43	4.79	1.54	0.12
	Not affected by fake news	83	3.59		
Anxiety	Affected by fake news	43	3.93	1.91	0.05
	Not affected by fake news	83	2.61		
Insomnia	Affected by fake news	43	10.86	1.88	0.05
	Not affected by fake news	83	8.66		

Regarding the specific questions related to the false news impact on the frontline medical staff, we obtained the following results: 34% of frontline healthcare workers answered yes to the question: "Are you affected by false news in the course of your professional activity?".

The most common answers to the question: "In what way fake news affects you?" were: "The doctor-patient relationship is affected. People distrust doctors and the medical system because they are misled by fake news." (23% of the respondents), "It affects me emotionally." (30% of the participants), and "It creates confusion." (19% of the respondents).

The top three words found in the answers of the frontline healthcare workers regarding the question: "What is the word that best describes the media position (print, audiovisual, online press) regarding medical staff during the outbreak of COVID-19?" are: "appreciation", (33% of the respondents), "distorted" (33% of the participants), and "objectivity" (15% of the respondents).

5. Discussion

The purpose of this research was to study if doctors and nurses who declared to be affected by false news show different types of psychological consequences than healthcare workers who do not consider themselves to be affected by fake news related to the COVID-19 pandemic.

The results were concordant with our predictions. Firstly, we found that almost half of the participants were affected by false news in their professional activity. The general population has been overwhelmed with information about COVID-19, including incorrect information and false information. Medical misinformation has centered around key themes: food and beverages as "cures," hygiene practices, and medicines. Healthcare workers must take action by refuting or rebutting misleading health information and providing appropriate information [16].

As false medical news about the novel coronavirus spread across the world, healthcare workers found themselves in another battle, the second pandemic, an infodemic. As one study shows, the job of healthcare workers has changed. Academics need to publicly denounce wrongdoers and hold them accountable with scientific evidence in the battle with fake news during the outbreak of COVID-19 [17].

The COVID-19 pandemic is putting health systems and healthcare workers around the world under immense pressure. Besides treating patients with COVID-19, medical specialists need to battle with another enemy, fake news. The frontline medical workers who declared to be affected by false news believe that misinformation affects them in many ways, such as: "I am emotionally affected by fake news.", "The doctor-patient relationship is affected by false medical news; patients distrust their doctors." "It consumes time and energy to battle misinformation. It creates confusion. "People are scared, and it takes more time and energy from our part to calm them and explain scientific information.", "Communication with patients influenced by fake news is difficult.", "It affects our professional reputation and credibility.", "It affects the general population's trust in the medical system and doctors. People who suffer from time-sensible health problems are afraid to go to hospitals to get treatment. That makes our job harder. It is sad and problematic for all of us, the healthcare workers."

Secondly, the frontline doctors and nurses who were declared to be affected by false news were significantly more stressed than healthcare workers who are not affected by medical misinformation related to the pandemic. Previous studies concerning the psychological sequelae observed during the SARS COV-1 in the 2003 outbreak revealed that healthcare workers experienced acute stress reactions [18]. In 2020, as one study shows, since the declaration of the coronavirus outbreak as a pandemic, some healthcare workers from different hospitals screened positive for moderate to extremely severe stress [19].

Work-associated stress affects healthcare workers, including doctors, nurses, auxiliary personnel, administrative staff, and other medical technicians. The three main work-related stress factors identified were: heavy workloads, the time-related pressure on the job, and extended working hours [20]. During a pandemic, frontline workers who are called upon to assist or treat those with COVID-19 may experience stress related to a physical strain of protective equipment, physical isolation, constant awareness, and vigilance regarding infection control procedures, pressures regarding procedures that must be followed [21]. Furthermore, as our study shows, frontline healthcare workers in Romania are influenced by false news and feel stress, among other psychological outcomes, in dealing with this particular factor concerning the public misinformation about the COVID-19 medical crisis.

Thirdly, the frontline medical workers who were declared to be affected by the infodemia felt more anxiety than healthcare workers who are not affected by false news related to pandemic time. The most frequently reported symptom during pandemic time is anxiety, both in the general population and medical staff. Many studies already demonstrated that frontline healthcare workers screened positive for moderate to severe anxiety during the outbreak of COVID-19. Before COVID-19, internet addiction was already recognized as a growing problem contributing to social anxiety, attention-deficit/hyperactivity disorder, and other wellness aspects, which may only intensify during a pandemic time [22].

Since the COVID-19 pandemic outbreak, the constant stream of information and fake medical news can be overwhelming for anyone, let alone clinicians already facing stressful challenges in their professional and personal lives [23]. False medical messages trigger feelings of fear and panic in public. When the message has an emotional impact, people are more inclined to share that information with family and friends. Despite our Government's efforts to communicate efficiently and disseminate medical information to the public, false news continued to spread much faster than the virus itself, leaving the medical community on the frontline of another battle, with misinformation and disinformation regarding the coronavirus crisis.

Finally, the frontline healthcare workers who are declared to be affected by misinformation suffer more from insomnia than healthcare workers who are not affected by false news related to pandemic time. Previous studies on emergency medicine specialists in Romania demonstrated that work-related stress symptoms, such as sleep disorders, play an essential role in the medical staff's mental health [24].

During a pandemic time, medical staff is placed under tremendous pressure, leading to many psychological reactions, including sleep disorders and low sleep quality, being present almost all the time [25,26]. A cross-sectional survey among healthcare workers treating patients with COVID-19 in China revealed that a significant proportion of participants experienced insomnia symptoms [27]. Having to face permanent dissemination of misinformation about the coronavirus, its treatments, evolution, impact, and even existence of the virus, the frontline medical workers felt the influence of this significant stress factor also, infodemia.

This research could be considered an initial attempt to integrate the false medical information stress-factor, among the other occupational stress causes during a pandemic time, which, to our understanding, is new and unique in Romanian frontline healthcare workers during the SARS COV-2 pandemic.

The results of this study should be evaluated, considering several limitations. One of the limits is the cross-sectional design. Our research cannot assess if there will be a change in variables over time. The relations found do not involve causal inferences between the studied variables. We attempted to compare the study groups concerning stress, depression, anxiety, and insomnia; further longitudinal research may contribute to a better understanding of ways in which the causality relationship regarding the false news effect on medical frontline healthcare workers and other psychological implications may occur. Another limit is the self-reported impact of the false news in the medical activity; the subjectivity of the cohort classification can be overcome in future research aiming at objective measurements of the false news factor. Despite the Romanian Strategic Communication Group's effort to present and explain in real-time, when possible, the false medical information that appeared in the Romanian media, separating false information from actual news can seem daunting and may influence our study variables.

Moreover, the sample size was too small. Further research with a larger sample, such as a nation-wide study, should be performed to gain a complete image of the fake news influence on doctors and nurses during the pandemic time. Longitudinal studies could further strengthen our conclusions and evidence of the relationships between fake news and different psychological outcomes Further research is needed to test a regression model of the study variables and factors that may be associated with the exposure to fake news in the medical and general population. Future research also may improve our knowledge of the impacts of false medical news, from efficient tools to discern between true and false content to better develop our cognitive reflection and overcome other psychological implications due to the exposure to false news in the COVID-19 pandemic.

6. Conclusions

In conclusion, our findings suggest that frontline healthcare workers who are declared to be affected by false news show different levels of psychological manifestations such as anxiety, stress, and insomnia, during the outbreak of the COVID-19 pandemic. They should be considered in the aftermath of the COVID-19 crisis when policies and interventions for positive mental health and well-being among frontline medical staff are designed and implemented.

Author Contributions: Conceptualization, I.S., D.V., L.M.B.; methodology, I.S., Z.P.C., D.V.; software, D.V.; validation, I.S., Z.P.C., D.V. and T.B.; formal analysis, D.V., T.B., L.M.B.; investigation, I.S., D.V.; resources, I.S., D.V., L.M.B.; data curation, I.S., D.V.; writing—original draft preparation, I.S., D.V.; writing—review and editing, I.S., D.V., T.B.; visualization, I.S., Z.P.C., D.V., T.B., L.M.B.; supervision, T.B.; project administration, I.S., D.V. All authors have read and agreed to the published version of the manuscript.

Funding: This research received no external funding.

Conflicts of Interest: The authors declare no conflict of interest.

Abbreviations

COVID 19	Coronavirus disease
WHO	World Health Organization
H1N1	Influenza A virus subtype H1N1
SARS COV2	Novel coronavirus
PPE	Personal protective equipment
The DASS-21	Depression, Anxiety and Stress Scale
SPSS	Statistical Package for Social Science

References

1. Gao, J.; Zheng, P.; Jia, Y.; Chen, H.; Mao, Y.; Chen, S.; Wang, Y.; Fu, H.; Dai, J. Mental health problems and social media exposure during COVID-19 outbreak. *PLoS ONE* **2020**, *15*, e0231924.
2. Depoux, A.; Martin, S.; Karafillakis, E.; Preet, R.; Wilder-Smith, A.; Larson, H. The pandemic of social media panic travels faster than the COVID-19 outbreak. *J. Travel Med.* **2020**, *27*, taaa031. [CrossRef] [PubMed]
3. Available online: https://www.nytimes.com/2020/02/06/health/coronavirus-misinformation-social-media.html (accessed on 7 July 2020).
4. Available online: https://www.merriam-webster.com/words-at-play/words-were-watching-infodemic-meaning (accessed on 25 June 2020).
5. Available online: https://www.who.int/campaigns/connecting-the-world-to-combat-coronavirus/how-to-report-misinformation-online (accessed on 30 October 2020).
6. Available online: https://www.un.org/en/un-coronavirus-communications-team/un-tackling-%E2%80%98infodemic%E2%80%99-misinformation-and-cybercrime-covid-19 (accessed on 15 July 2020).
7. Chew, C.; Eysenbach, G. Pandemics in the Age of Twitter: Content Analysis of Tweets during the 2009 H1N1 Outbreak. *PLoS ONE* **2010**, *5*, e14118. [CrossRef] [PubMed]
8. Raghuvir, K.; Anila, A.; Ganesh, N.P.; Jayesh, M.; Krishnadas, N. COVID-19: Emergence, Spread, Possible Treatments, and Global Burden. *Front. Public Health* **2020**, *8*, 216.
9. Torales, J.; O'Higgins, M.; Castaldelli-Maia, J.M.; Ventriglio, A. The outbreak of COVID-19 coronavirus and its impact on global mental health. *Int. J. Soc. Psychiatry* **2020**, *66*, 317–320. [CrossRef] [PubMed]
10. Available online: https://newseu.cgtn.com/news/2020-04-11/How-are-healthcare-workers-coping-with-fighting-COVID-19--PBrX22rp6w/index.html (accessed on 15 July 2020).
11. Chew, N.; Lee, G.; Tan, B.; Jing, M.; Goh, Y.; Ngiam, N.; Yeo, L.; Ahmad, A.; Ahmed Khan, F.; Shanmugam, G.N.; et al. A multinational, multicentre study on the psychological outcomes and associated physical symptoms amongst healthcare workers during COVID-19 outbreak. *Brain Behav. Immun.* **2020**, *88*, 559–565. [CrossRef] [PubMed]
12. Available online: http://legislatie.just.ro/Public/DetaliiDocument/224501 (accessed on 15 July 2020).
13. Secosan, I.; Virga, D.; Crainiceanu, Z.P.; Bratu, T. The Mediating Role of Insomnia and Exhaustion in the Relationship between Secondary Traumatic Stress and Mental Health Complaints among Frontline Medical Staff during the COVID-19 Pandemic. *Behav. Sci.* **2020**, *10*, 164. [CrossRef] [PubMed]
14. Zanon, C.; Brenner, R.E.; Baptista, M.N.; Vogel, D.L.; Rubin, M.; Al-Darmaki, F.R.; Gonçalves, M.; Heath, P.J.; Liao, H.-Y.; MacKenzie, C.S.; et al. Examining the Dimensionality, Reliability, and Invariance of the Depression, Anxiety, and Stress Scale–21 (DASS-21) Across Eight Countries. *Assessment* **2020**. [CrossRef] [PubMed]

15. Morin, C.M.; Belleville, G.; Bélanger, L.; Ivers, H. The Insomnia Severity Index: Psychometric Indicators to Detect Insomnia Cases and Evaluate Treatment Response. *Sleep* **2011**, *34*, 601–608. [CrossRef] [PubMed]
16. Cathal, O.C.; Michelle, M. Going viral: Doctors must tackle fake news in the covid-19 pandemic. *BMJ* **2020**, *369*, m1587.
17. Tapia, L. COVID-19 and Fake News in the Dominican Republic. *Am. J. Trop. Med. Hyg.* **2020**, *102*, 1172–1174. [CrossRef] [PubMed]
18. Tam, C.W.C.; Pang, E.P.F.; Lam, L.C.W.; Chiu, H.F.K. Severe acute respiratory syndrome (SARS) in Hong Kong in 2003: Stress and psychological impact among frontline healthcare workers. *Psychol. Med.* **2020**, *34*, 1197–1204. [CrossRef] [PubMed]
19. Elbay, R.Y.; Kurtulmuş, A.; Arpacıoğlu, S.; Karadere, E. Depression, anxiety, stress levels of physicians and associated factors in Covid-19 pandemics. *Psychiatry Res.* **2020**, *290*, 113130. [CrossRef] [PubMed]
20. Tsai, Y.; Liu, C. Factors and symptoms associated with work stress and health-promoting lifestyles among hospital staff: A pilot study in Taiwan. *BMC Health Serv. Res.* **2012**, *12*, 199. [CrossRef] [PubMed]
21. Available online: https://www.ptsd.va.gov/covid/COVID19ManagingStressHCW032020.pdf (accessed on 15 July 2020).
22. Weinstein, A.; Lejoyeux, M. Internet addiction or excessive internet use. *Am. J. Drug Alcohol Abus.* **2010**, *36*, 277–283. [CrossRef] [PubMed]
23. Bansal, P.; Bingemann, T.A.; Greenhawt, M.; Mosnaim, G.; Nanda, A.; Oppenheimer, J.; Sharma, H.; Stukus, D.; Shaker, M. Clinician Wellness During the COVID-19 Pandemic: Extraordinary Times and Unusual Challenges for the Allergist/Immunologist. *J. Allergy Clin. Immunol. Pract.* **2020**, *8*, 1781–1790.e3. [CrossRef] [PubMed]
24. Secosan, I.; Bredicean, C.; Crainiceanu, Z.P.; Virga, D.; Giurgi-Oncu, C.; Bratu, T. Mental Health in Emergency Medical Clinicians: Burnout, STS, Sleep Disorders. A Cross-Sectional Descriptive Multicentric Study. *Cent. Eur. Ann. Clin. Res.* **2019**, *1*, 12–16. [CrossRef]
25. Maunder, R.; Hunter, J.; Vincent, L.; Bennett, J.; Peladeau, N.; Leszcz, M.; Sadavoy, J.; Verhaeghe, L.M.; Steinberg, R.; Mazzulli, T. The immediate psychological and occupational impact of the 2003 SARS outbreak in a teaching hospital. *CMAJ* **2003**, *168*, 1245–1251. [PubMed]
26. Chen, R.; Chou, K.R.; Huang, Y.J.; Wang, T.S.; Liu, S.Y.; Ho, L.Y. Effects of a SARS prevention programme in Taiwan on nursing staff's anxiety, depression and sleep quality: A longitudinal survey. *Int. J. Nurs. Stud.* **2006**, *43*, 215–225. [CrossRef] [PubMed]
27. Lai, J.; Ma, S.; Wang, Y.; Cai, Z.; Hu, J.; Wei, N.; Wu, J.; Du, H.; Chen, T.; Li, R.; et al. Factors Associated With Mental Health Outcomes Among Health Care Workers Exposed to Coronavirus Disease 2019. *JAMA Netw. Open* **2020**, *3*, e203976. [CrossRef]

Publisher's Note: MDPI stays neutral with regard to jurisdictional claims in published maps and institutional affiliations.

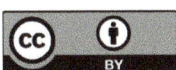

© 2020 by the authors. Licensee MDPI, Basel, Switzerland. This article is an open access article distributed under the terms and conditions of the Creative Commons Attribution (CC BY) license (http://creativecommons.org/licenses/by/4.0/).

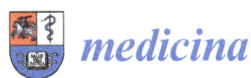

Article

Evaluation of Different Positive End-Expiratory Pressures Using Supreme™ Airway Laryngeal Mask during Minor Surgical Procedures in Children

Mascha O. Fiedler [1,*], Elisabeth Schätzle [2], Marius Contzen [3], Christian Gernoth [4], Christel Weiß [5], Thomas Walter [6], Tim Viergutz [2] and Armin Kalenka [7]

1. Clinic of Anesthesiology, Heidelberg University Hospital, 69120 Heidelberg, Germany
2. Clinic of Anesthesiology and Surgical Intensive Care Medicine, University Medical Centre Mannheim, 68167 Mannheim, Germany; eb.schaetzle@gmx.de (E.S.); tim.viergutz@umm.de (T.V.)
3. Department of Anesthesiology and Intensive Care Medicine, Heilig-Geist-Hospital Bensheim, 64625 Bensheim, Germany; marius.contzen@artemed.de
4. Department of Anesthesiology, Surgical Intensive Care Medicine, Pain Therapy, Helios Hospital Duisburg, 47166 Duisburg, Germany; christian.gernoth@helios-gesundheit.de
5. Department of Medical Statistics, University Medical Centre Mannheim, 68167 Mannheim, Germany; christel.weiss@medma.uni-heidelberg.de
6. Emergency Department, University Medical Centre Mannheim, 68167 Mannheim, Germany; thomas.walter.med@umm.de
7. Department of Anesthesiology and Intensive Care Medicine, Hospital Bergstrasse, 64646 Heppenheim, Germany; armin.kalenka@kkh-bergstrasse.de
* Correspondence: mascha.fiedler@med.uni-heidelberg.de; Tel.: +49-(0)-6222-1563-9434

Received: 21 September 2020; Accepted: 19 October 2020; Published: 21 October 2020

Abstract: *Background and objectives:* The laryngeal mask is the method of choice for airway management in children during minor surgical procedures. There is a paucity of data regarding optimal management of mechanical ventilation in these patients. The Supreme™ airway laryngeal mask offers the option to insert a gastric tube to empty the stomach contents of air and/or gastric juice. The aim of this investigation was to evaluate the impact of positive end-expiratory positive pressure (PEEP) levels on ventilation parameters and gastric air insufflation during general anesthesia in children using pressure-controlled ventilation with laryngeal mask. *Materials and Methods:* An observational trial was carried out in 67 children aged between 1 and 11 years. PEEP levels of 0, 3 and 5 mbar were tested for 5 min in each patient during surgery and compared with ventilation parameters (dynamic compliance (mL/cmH$_2$O), etCO$_2$ (mmHg), peak pressure (mbar), tidal volume (mL), respiratory rate (per minute), FiO$_2$ and gastric air (mL)) were measured at each PEEP. Air was aspirated from the stomach at the start of the sequence of measurements and at the end. *Results:* Significant differences were observed for the ventilation parameters: dynamic compliance (PEEP 5 vs. PEEP 3: $p < 0.0001$, PEEP 5 vs. PEEP 0: $p < 0.0001$, PEEP 3 vs. PEEP 0: $p < 0.0001$), peak pressure (PEEP 5 vs. PEEP 3: $p < 0.0001$, PEEP 5 vs. PEEP 0: $p < 0.0001$, PEEP 3 vs. PEEP 0: $p < 0.0001$) and tidal volume (PEEP 5 vs. PEEP 3: $p = 0.0048$, PEEP 5 vs. PEEP 0: $p < 0.0001$, PEEP 3 vs. PEEP 0: $p < 0.0001$). All parameters increased significantly with higher PEEP, with the exception of etCO$_2$ (significant decrease) and respiratory rate (no significant difference). We also showed different values for air quantity in the comparisons between the different PEEP levels (PEEP 5: 2.8 ± 3.9 mL, PEEP 3: 1.8 ± 3.0 mL; PEEP 0: 1.6 ± 2.3 mL) with significant differences between PEEP 5 and PEEP 3 ($p = 0.0269$) and PEEP 5 and PEEP 0 ($p = 0.0209$). *Conclusions:* Our data suggest that ventilation with a PEEP of 5 mbar might be more lung protective in children using the Supreme™ airway laryngeal mask, although gastric air insufflation increased with higher PEEP. We recommend the use of a laryngeal mask with the option of inserting a gastric tube to evacuate potential gastric air.

Keywords: paediatric anaesthesia; laryngeal mask; gastric insufflation; PEEP; airway devices; respiratory function

1. Introduction

The laryngeal mask is a well-established option for airway management in pediatric patients undergoing general anesthesia for various surgeries [1]. This device can be used to secure ventilation in difficult situations, for example, after primary failure of endotracheal intubation [2–4].

Laryngeal mask airway (LMA) provides a relatively safe airway for positive pressure ventilation (PPV) in children [5]. Pressure control ventilation (PCV) is widely discussed as the method of choice for delivery of PPV through an LMA. A study by Natalini et al. compared pressure-controlled ventilation and volume-controlled ventilation with the LMA. The study demonstrated that the use of PCV during general anesthesia with the LMA reduced the peak airway pressure compared with volume control ventilation at the same tidal volumes and inspiratory times [6]. Positive end-expiratory pressure (PEEP) is frequently used in tracheally intubated patients to increase oxygenation, but is rarely used with the LMA because the low pressure seal predisposes to oropharyngeal and esophageal air leaks [7].

The use of general anesthetic reduces functional residual capacity especially in children, resulting in increased intrapulmonary shunts [8]. PEEP reduces this shunt volume during controlled ventilation in patients with healthy lungs [9]. There are no guidelines for PEEP settings in pediatric patients. Nevertheless, anesthesiologists traditionally set PEEP to a lower level in pediatric patients than in adults, i.e., below 5 cmH$_2$O [8].

Optimization of functional residual capacity is even more important in children since they have a lower capacity for elastic retraction and a lower relaxation volume, and as a result are more susceptible to atelectasis than adults [10]. However, there is little data on optimum ventilation using a laryngeal mask and applying PEEP.

The Supreme™ laryngeal mask (S-LMA, a second-generation laryngeal mask) offers the option of simultaneous insertion of a gastric tube. This is important as, in contrast to airway management using endotracheal intubation, use of a laryngeal mask is potentially associated with the risk of gastric air insufflation with possible further consequences. But a randomized controlled trial by Drake-Brockman et al. evaluated the effect of endotracheal tubes versus LMAs on perioperative respiratory adverse events (PRAE) in infants [11]. The primary outcome of this study was the incidence of any PRAE in relation to the type of airway device used. The impact of LMA vs. endotracheal tubes (ETT) on the incidence of individual PRAE and their timing (intraoperatively and postoperatively) were assessed as secondary outcomes. This study showed a clear benefit of the use of an LMA compared with an endotracheal tube in a large number of infants undergoing minor elective surgery.

The aim of our observational investigation was to evaluate the effects on ventilation parameters during general anesthesia in children using pressure-controlled ventilation with the S-LMA at different PEEP levels. Primary outcome parameters were changes of the dynamic compliance and end-tidal carbon dioxide (etCO$_2$) to verify recruitment maneuver's with PEEP in lungs; secondary outcome parameters were the gastric air insufflation during ventilation with three different PEEP levels.

2. Methods

This prospective clinical trial was carried out from February 2012 to August 2014. Included children were aged between 1 and 11 years old, with American Society of Anaesthesiologists (ASA) classification I-III, scheduled for a minor elective surgery (inguinal hernia repair or circumcision) under general anesthesia in supine position with a planned surgery duration <30 min. Inclusion of patients was after informed consent. The study protocol was been approved by the Medical Ethics Committee II of the Mannheim Medical Faculty of the University of Heidelberg (2010-264N-MA; 22 June 2010).

Exclusion criteria were an ASA classification of IV and above, children with known difficult airways or impossibility of insertion of the laryngeal mask or the gastric tube. The size of the S-LMA (Teleflex Medical Europe Ltd., Athlone, Ireland) (see Table 1), the gastric tube and the cuff filling volume were selected based on weight-adapted tables provided by the manufacturer [12]. The cuff was inflated to a recommended maximum of 60 cmH$_2$O using a cuff pressure monitor [12,13].

Table 1. Baseline characteristics.

Characteristic			All Patients ($n = 67$)
Age, year			4.7 ± 2.4
Range			1.1–10.8
Gender	n (%)		
Male			55 (82)
Female			12 (18)
Body weight *, kg			
			19.5 ± 8.4
Range, kg			9–59
Groups *	n (%)		
	<5 kg	Supreme™ laryngeal mask size (1)	0 (0)
	5–10 kg	Supreme™ laryngeal mask size (1.5)-	5 (8)
	10–20 kg	Supreme™ laryngeal mask size (2)	38 (58)
	20–30 kg	Supreme™ laryngeal mask size (2.5)	17 (26)
	30–50 kg	Supreme™ laryngeal mask size (3)	5 (8)
	50–70 kg	Supreme™ laryngeal mask size (4)	1 (2)

* Information on body weight was unavailable for one subject.

A total of 71 children were included in the study (ASA class I or II, all without lung disease). In two children investigation was stopped due to a leakage of the laryngeal mask and in two other children investigation had to be discontinued because the gastric tube could not be positioned for adequate function. These four children were excluded from the statistical analysis. Thus, the data for 67 children (12 girls and 55 boys) were available for final analysis.

2.1. General Anaesthesia

Each child was given premedication with midazolam (Dormicum®, Roche Pharma, Grenzach-Wyhlen, Germany) (0.5 mg/kg bodyweight (bw)) per os within 30 min of induction of anesthesia.

Balanced or total intravenous anesthesia was used. Each patient was connected to a Dräger Primus® (Drägerwerk, Lübeck, Germany) machine. Standard monitors included precordial stethoscope, pulse oximeter, electrocardiography, automated noninvasive blood pressure (NIBP), capnometer and nasopharyngeal temperature.

The subject was pre-oxygenated with an inspiratory oxygen fraction of 80% and 4 L fresh gas flow per minute using a facemask. Thereafter we administered 2–4 µg fentanyl (Fentanyl Janssen®, Jansen-Cilag, Neuss, Germany) per kilogram bw and 4–6 mg propofol 10 mg/mL (Propofol®, Fresenius Kabi, Bad Homburg, Germany) per kilogram bw via a previously inserted intravenous cannula. Muscle relaxants were not required at any point during the investigation.

We did not perform bag-valve mask ventilation. The subject was pre-oxygenated and after the administration of fentanyl and propofol we inserted the S-LMA. At this time point, no monitoring of gastric air insufflation was undertaken. Lidocaine gel (Xylocain Gel 2%, Astra Zeneca, Wedel, Germany) recommended as a lubricant by the manufacturer [12], was applied to the back of the S-LMA prior to insertion. Adequate ventilation was verified based on the gel displacement test [12,14], bilaterally visible respiratory excursion, bilateral auscultation of the breath sounds and capnography.

A leakage test was carried out after the laryngeal mask had been fixed in place and connected to the ventilator. This was the airway pressure generated when an audible noise was heard over the mouth. Airway leak pressure was measured beforehand at a minimum pressure of 18 cmH$_2$O and a maximum pressure of 25 cmH$_2$O. We excluded patients from our study if the airway leak pressure was under the minimum pressure.

Pressure-controlled ventilation was carried out with a tidal volume of 6 to 8 mL/kg bw and a PEEP of 3 mbar. The inspiratory oxygen fraction (F$_i$O$_2$) was reduced from 80% to 50%, aiming at an oxygen saturation of above 95% and an end-tidal carbon dioxide (etCO$_2$) concentration of 33–39 mmHg. A balanced anesthesia was maintained to the end of the surgery, using sevofluran (Sevofluran Baxter, Baxter, Unterschleißheim, Germany) with a minimal alveolar concentration (MAC) of 0.8, or as a total intravenous anesthesia using propofol. The equilibration period was not defined.

After positioning of the S-LMA, each patient received a lubricated gastric tube through the drainage canal. Measurement time started after the insertion of the gastric tube and the withdrawal of the contents of the stomach (fluids or air) with a 5 mL syringe.

2.2. Data Collection

The recorded ventilation parameters included the dynamic compliance, etCO$_2$, peak inspiratory pressure (PIP), inspiration volume, respiratory rate (RR), and the FiO$_2$ for each PEEP level. Additionally, gastric air and aspirates/secretions were documented. We did not measure the BMI of the children and we didn't take the time of the surgery during our measurements.

Once anesthesia was established, PEEP was increased to 5 mbar for 5 min (T0), PEEP was then reduced to 3 mbar for 5 min (T1) and to 0 mbar for 5 min (T2). Peak inspiration pressure was kept constant during all PEEP levels. All measurements were performed during the surgical procedure. The patients were not breathing spontaneously. The laryngeal mask was removed correctly at the end of surgery once the patient was awake and exhibiting sufficient spontaneous respiration and an adequate presence of protective reflexes.

2.3. Statistical Analysis

Statistical analysis was carried out using the statistical software package SAS, release 9.4 (SAS Institute, Cary, NC, USA).

Quantitative variables are presented as mean and standard deviation together with their range (see Table 1). Data approximately normally distributed (i.e., dynamic compliance, etCO$_2$, peak pressure, tidal volume, respiratory rate) that had been recorded multiple times for a given observation unit was analyzed using repeated measures ANOVA. The SAS procedure PROC MIXED with the fixed factors "measuring point", patients' age and body weight group and the random factor "patient ID" was used for this purpose based on three defined PEEP levels (T0: PEEP 5, T1: PEEP 3 and T2: PEEP 0 mbar).

To compare gastric air at different time points the Friedman test was used, since this parameter may not be considered normally distributed. For pairwise comparisons of measurement time points, post hoc tests according to Scheffé or Wilcoxon test for 2 paired samples were used, respectively. The result of a statistical test was considered as significant for $p < 0.05$.

3. Results

Baseline characteristics are presented in Table 1. The youngest child was aged 13 months and the oldest 10 years and 10 months. Mean body weight was 19.5 ± 8.4 kg.

3.1. Ventilation Parameters

Comparison of RR, tidal volume (V$_t$), peak pressure, dynamic compliance, expiratory carbon dioxide concentration (etCO$_2$), inspiratory oxygen fraction (FiO$_2$) and quantity of gastric air at T0 (PEEP 5 mbar), T1 (PEEP 3 mbar) and T2 (PEEP 0 mbar) are shown in Table 2.

Table 2. Ventilation parameters and gastric air by PEEP.

	T0 (PEEP 5) (mbar)	T1 (PEEP 3) (mbar)	T2 (PEEP 0) (mbar)	p-Values for Pairwise Comparisons
Dynamic compliance C_{dyn} (mL/cmH$_2$O)	18.4 ± 7.5	16.8 ± 6.9	14.4 ± 5.5	T0-T1: <0.0001 T0-T2: <0.0001 T1-T2: <0.0001
etCO$_2$ (mmHg)	37.1 ± 4.7	38.2 ± 4.3	41.3 ± 5.1	T0-T2: <0.0001 T1-T2: <0.0001
Peak pressure (mbar)	14.9 ± 1.6	13.0 ± 1.6	10.6 ± 1.5	T0-T1: <0.0001 T0-T2: <0.0001 T1-T2: <0.0001
V_t (mL)	170.4 ± 66.2	160.2 ± 60.8	138.8 ± 50.2	T0-T1: 0.0048 T0-T2: <0.0001 T1-T2: <0.0001
RR (per minute)	20.9 ± 3.8	20.9 ± 3.8	21.0 ± 3.8	not significant
FiO$_2$	0.51 ± 0.06	0.49 ± 0.06	0.49 ± 0.06	not significant
Gastric air (mL)	2.8 ± 3.9	1.8 ± 3.0	1.6 ± 2.43	T0-T1: 0.0269 T0-T2: 0.0209

For each PEEP level—with the only exception of respiratory rate, $p = 0.3708$—changes over time could be detected (each $p < 0.0001$) (Table 2).

There was a significant decrease in dynamic compliance as PEEP levels reduced (PEEP 5 > PEEP 3 > PEEP 0).

A significant increase in etCO$_2$ concentration was observed with decreasing PEEP (PEEP 5 < PEEP 3 < PEEP 0). The inspiratory oxygen fraction (FiO$_2$) was not significant.

The mean airway leak pressure was 22.5 ± 2 cmH$_2$O.

3.2. Gastric Air or Aspirates/Secretion

An important endpoint of our study was the amount of gastric air or aspirates during mechanical ventilation with S-LMA and three different PEEP levels.

Also, for this parameter, changes over time have been found ($p = 0.0176$). Wilcoxon tests for two paired samples revealed significant differences between PEEP 5 and PEEP 3 ($p = 0.0269$) as well as PEEP 5 and PEEP 0 ($p = 0.0209$). We did not aspirate any gastric secretion.

4. Discussion

The principal findings of the present observational clinical trial are that a PEEP of 5 mbar provides significantly higher dynamic compliance (C_{dyn}), tidal volume (V_t) and peak pressure during general anesthesia in children using PCV with the S-LMA at different PEEP levels. We also found a significantly higher gastric air volume during ventilation with a PEEP of 5 mbar.

The S-LMA with the additional option of insertion of a gastric tube was used in this investigation of different PEEP levels during minor elective surgical interventions in children. We used this S-LMA because with the opportunity of insertion of a gastric tube during PCV and the application with PEEP, the insufflation of air and the risk of aspiration seems to be higher.

According to several studies, sufficient PEEP should be used to minimize atelectasis and maintain oxygenation [5,9,15,16]. Serafini et al. examined ten children, ranged from ages 1 to 3 years, all without lung disease. After general anesthesia for cranial or abdominal CT scans, pulmonary morphology was investigated. A PEEP of 5 cmH$_2$O was shown to recruit all available alveolar units and to induce the disappearance of atelectasis in dependent lung regions [17]. However, after full muscle relaxation, ventilation was with an orotracheal tube and not with a laryngeal mask in this study.

Our study demonstrated that without muscle relaxation the children might develop atelectasis, and that ventilation with S-LMA and PEEP of 5 mbar improves the dynamic compliance and recruited the lungs.

Goldmann and colleagues tested the hypothesis that in anaesthetized pediatric patients the ProSeal™ laryngeal mask (P-LMA) can be used effectively to apply a PEEP of 5 cmH_2O during pressure-controlled ventilation (PCV) and that this leads to an improved arterial oxygenation compared to a PCV ventilation without PEEP [18]. It seems that the application of PEEP (5 cmH_2O) during PCV improves gas exchange in healthy pediatric patients [18]. We did not take arterial blood gas samples in our setting. The duration of minor surgeries in our setting was not as long as the procedures in the study from Goldman et al.

A randomized controlled trial with 90 children showed that PCV with PEEP using the P-LMA was accompanied with lower incidence of adverse events in comparison to spontaneous respiration in infants and toddlers with upper respiratory tract infection undergoing infra umbilical surgeries under general anesthesia. The authors concluded that PCV with PEEP using P-LMA may be the preferred mode of ventilation in children [19].

In our study, we found significant differences in C_{dyn} through different PEEP levels during PCV. C_{dyn} was significantly greater for a PEEP of 5 mbar. In pediatric patients PEEP is traditionally set lower, but we have not found profound reasoning in the literature, empirically, anesthesiologists tend to ventilate children with a lower PEEP compared to adult patients. Wirth et al. investigated whether moderately higher PEEP improves respiratory mechanics and regional ventilation. Therefore, 40 children were mechanically ventilated with PEEP 2 and 5 cmH_2O. They analyzed volume-dependent compliance profiles as a measure of intratidal recruitment/derecruitment. They concluded that increasing PEEP from 2 to 5 cmH_2O improved mean compliance and was associated with improved peripheral ventilation without causing overdistension of the lungs or hemodynamic compromise [8]. This was the first study investigating the effects of PEEP on intratidal compliance in children. Compared to our study children received full neuromuscular block, they did a tracheal intubation during anesthesia and invasive ventilation and the planned surgery duration was >60 min.

In a study by von Ungern-Sternberg et al. [10], younger children were more susceptible to atelectasis than older children and benefited from higher PEEP settings. Another study in children showed that increasing the PEEP can reopen dorsal areas of the lungs [17]. As the closing capacity is lower at younger age, younger children have a higher probability that closing capacity is lower than FRC (functional residual capacity). As a consequence, small airways tend to collapse at the end of expiration. Therefore, particularly in younger children a higher PEEP might be required to shift FRC to a level at which the collapse of the small airways is prevented [8,10].

Furthermore, we demonstrated in our study that the behavior of $etCO_2$ concentration opposed that of C_{dyn}. $EtCO_2$ concentration was significantly higher at a PEEP of 0 mbar than at 5 mbar. This is possibly due to the higher C_{dyn} arising from the larger gas exchange area (recruitment with PEEP and minute volume), whereby the carbon dioxide is more easily exhaled.

In our study, we posed the question of whether increasing the PEEP level results in an increase in the rate of gastric air insufflation during ventilation with S-LMA. The analyses revealed that there were significant differences in the quantities of gastric air obtained via the gastric tube for the different PEEP levels in the overall data analysis. Lagarde et al. noted in their study that the incidence of gastric air insufflation rises with increasing inspiratory pressure under face mask ventilation [20]. The ventilation with a face mask for further pre-oxygenation prior to positioning of the S-LMA is probably the reason for positive quantities of air. Therefore, we did not ventilate each child during pre-oxygenation with the mask.

We also recorded in our study the highest peak pressure with a PEEP of 5 mbar merely around 15 mbar and significant reduction of the gastric air quantity with the decrease of the PEEP levels. Lagarde et al. describe gastric air insufflation in children as occurring in over 58% at an inspiratory pressure of above 15 cmH_2O [20]. However, gastric air insufflation was detected through auscultation of the stomach in this experimental setup. How high the rates for false positives and negatives were in this study is unclear. According to the literature, gastric air insufflation occurs at an earlier stage in younger subjects than in older ones. A limit of below 15 cmH$_2$O for inspiratory pressure and, in some cases even below 10 cmH$_2$O, is referred for children below the age of one year. The inspiratory pressure therefore appears to be age-dependent [20]. Bouvet et al. reach the conclusion that an inspiratory pressure of 15 cmH$_2$O is probably the best compromise between adequate ventilation with a face mask and gastric air insufflation [21]. However, PEEP is not used in this study and the reduced incidence of gastric air insufflation is related to the induction phase of anesthesia [21]. The probability of gastric air insufflation arises due to the use of PCV, as this results in lower inspiratory pressures for volume-controlled ventilation at the same tidal volume. The inspiratory pressure of 15 cmH$_2$O is recommended as the standard limit in children as no further increase in tidal volume is achieved and there is an increased incidence of gastric air insufflation above this value [20]. The correct positioning of the airway device, such as the laryngeal mask, appears to be the decisive factor in achieving optimum sealing and avoiding any potential axial rotation, thereby ensuring that less air enters the stomach [22,23].

A further question that arises repeatedly is whether insufflation of air increases the patients' risk of aspiration.

The results of our investigation showed a tendency that the quantity of the gastric air can be reduced following aspiration through the gastric tube in the S-LMA. Maybe the opportunity of a gastric tube can lower the risk of regurgitation and aspiration.

However, the precise reduction in the risk of aspiration cannot be derived from our available data. In a retrospective analysis, Bernadini et al. demonstrated that, compared to an endotracheal tube, there is no increase in the risk of aspiration when using a laryngeal mask, but that the majority of cases of aspiration occurred in patients who required emergency surgery [24].

Our investigation was subject to some limitations. The patients included in this study were aged between 1 year and 11 years. The range of age is very large and consequently the group is heterogenous (weight and height). Therefore, the results obtained in the present investigation cannot be directly extrapolated to younger children and certainly not to older children or even adults. To minimize the risk of complications, only children with uncomplicated airways were investigated. Furthermore, this is not a blinded study as no experimental and control groups were formed. A critical view must also be taken in relation to the short duration of 5 min for the application of PEEP. It might be possible to obtain more clear-cut results if both the individual PEEPs were tested for longer periods and a greater overall number of subjects with a better age distribution were to be investigated. The range of different PEEP levels were very small. In our study, the focus was set on these levels because pediatric anesthetists are used to lower PEEP levels.

We also used only one kind of laryngeal mask with the advantage of a channel for a gastric tube. Additionally, the amount of gastric air should better be evaluated by gastric ultrasound or auscultation, a method well established in anesthesia practice today. The evacuation of gastric air over the gastric tube by aspiration via a syringe is not as valid as gastric ultrasound. This is a limitation of our study and we need further randomized investigations with more patients to figure out the risk of aspiration during ventilation with laryngeal masks.

5. Conclusions

Our results revealed that a higher PEEP, maximum 5 mbar in our investigation, yielded more ventilator-associated advantages than disadvantages with the S-LMA. Results on this were usually significant, especially for a PEEP of 5 mbar, with a larger inspiration volume, greater C_{dyn} and a lower etCO$_2$ concentration.

Our investigation also demonstrates that significant quantities of air are insufflate into the stomach under PCV with the S-LMA and a PEEP of up to 5 mbar.

However, it must be noted, that air was collected mainly after induction of anesthesia and ventilation with the S-LMA after insertion of this device. The question therefore arises, as to whether routine aspiration of air from the stomach significantly reduces the incidence of aspiration when the S-LMA, and possibly also other supraglottic airway devices, are used. This could constitute a hypothesis for future studies with a larger sample size.

Overall, the conclusion can at least be drawn that a positive PEEP value is more suitable than no PEEP during ventilation with S-LMA in children.

Author Contributions: Conceptualization, M.O.F., T.V., M.C. and C.G.; methodology, T.V., M.C., C.G.; software, C.W.; validation, C.W., E.S. and M.O.F.; formal analysis, C.W.; investigation, E.S.; resources, T.V.; data curation, C.W., A.K.; writing—original draft preparation, M.O.F.; writing—review and editing, M.O.F., E.S., C.W., T.W., T.V., A.K.; visualization, E.S., C.W.; supervision, A.K.; project administration, T.V.; funding acquisition, T.V. All authors have read and agreed to the published version of the manuscript.

Funding: The study was financed by the University Medical Centre Mannheim.

Acknowledgments: We would like to acknowledge our colleagues from the department of anesthesiology of the University Medical Centre of Mannheim for their collaboration. We want to thank the parents of our research for their support and for all of the opportunities we were given to further our research.

Conflicts of Interest: The authors report no conflict of interest.

Ethical Approval: The study protocol has been approved by the Medical Ethics Committee II of the Mannheim Medical Faculty of the University of Heidelberg (2010-264N-MA; 22 June 2010) and registered at the German Clinical Trails Register (DRKS00013254).

References

1. Jain, R.A.; Parikh, D.A.; Malde, A.D. Balasubramanium, B. Current practice patterns of supraglottic airway device usage in paediatric patients amongst anaesthesiologists: A nationwide survey. *Indian J. Anaesth.* **2018**, *62*, 269–279. [PubMed]
2. Goyal, R. Small is the new big: An overview of newer supraglottic airways for children. *J. Anaesthesiol. Clin. Pharmacol.* **2015**, *31*, 440–449. [CrossRef] [PubMed]
3. Jagannathan, N.; Sequera-Ramos, L.; Sohn, L.; Wallis, B.; Shertzer, A.; Schaldenbrand, K. Elective use of supraglottic airway devices for primary airway management in children with difficult airways. *Br. J. Anaesth.* **2014**, *112*, 742–748. [CrossRef] [PubMed]
4. Asai, T.; Nagata, A.; Shingu, K. Awake tracheal intubation through the laryngeal mask in neonates with upper airway obstruction. *Paediatr. Anaesth.* **2008**, *18*, 77–80. [CrossRef]
5. Gursoy, F.; Algren, J.T.; Skjonsby, B.S. Positive pressure ventilation with the laryngeal mask airway in children. *Anesth. Analg.* **1996**, *82*, 33–38.
6. Natalini, G.; Facchetti, P.; Dicembrini, M.A.; Lanza, G.; Rosano, A.; Bernardini, A. Pressure controlled versus volume controlled ventilation with laryngeal mask airway. *J. Clin. Anesth.* **2001**, *13*, 436–439. [CrossRef]
7. Von Goedecke, A.; Brimacombe, J.; Keller, C.; Hoermann, C.; Loeckinger, A.; Rieder, J.; Kleinsasser, A. Positive pressure versus pressure support ventilation at different levels of PEEP using the ProSeal laryngeal mask airway. *Anaesth. Intensive Care* **2004**, *32*, 804–808. [CrossRef]
8. Wirth, S.; Artner, L.; Bross, T.; Lozano-Zahonero, S.; Spaeth, J.; Schumann, S. Intratidal recruitment/derecruitment persists at low and moderate positive end-expiratory pressure in paediatric patients. *Respir. Physiol. Neurobiol.* **2016**, *234*, 9–13. [CrossRef]
9. Imberger, G.; McIlroy, D.; Pace, N.L.; Wetterslev, J.; Brok, J.; Moller, A.M. Positive end-expiratory pressure (PEEP) during anaesthesia for the prevention of mortality and postoperative pulmonary complications. *Cochrane Database Syst. Rev.* **2010**, *9*, CD007922. [CrossRef]

10. Von Ungern-Sternberg, B.S.; Regli, A.; Schibler, A.; Hammer, J.; Frei, F.J.; Erb, T.O. The impact of positive end-expiratory pressure on functional residual capacity and ventilation homogeneity impairment in anesthetized children exposed to high levels of inspired oxygen. *Anesth. Analg.* **2007**, *104*, 1364–1368. [CrossRef]
11. Drake-Brockman, T.F.; Ramgolam, A.; Zhang, G.; Hall, G.L.; Von Ungern-Sternberg, B.S. The effect of endotracheal tubes versus laryngeal mask airways on perioperative respiratory adverse events in infants: A randomised controlled trial. *Lancet* **2017**, *389*, 701–708. [CrossRef]
12. Instructions for Use—LMA Supreme. 2015. Available online: http://www.lmaco-ifu.com/sites/default/files/node/438/ifu/revision/3593/ifu-lma-supreme-paj2100002buk.pdf (accessed on 24 February 2015).
13. Choi, K.W.; Lee, J.R.; Oh, J.T.; Kim, D.W.; Kim, M.S. The randomized crossover comparison of airway sealing with the laryngeal mask airway Supreme at three different intracuff pressures in children. *Paediatr. Anaesth.* **2014**, *24*, 1080–1087. [CrossRef] [PubMed]
14. Sharma, B.; Sood, J.; Sahai, C.; Kumra, V.P. Troubleshooting ProSeal LMA. *Indian J. Anaesth.* **2009**, *53*, 414–424. [PubMed]
15. Feldman, J.M. Optimal ventilation of the anesthetized pediatric patient. *Anesth. Analg.* **2015**, *120*, 165–175. [CrossRef] [PubMed]
16. Goldmann, K. Clinical basics of supraglottic airway management in paediatric anaesthesia. *Anasthesiol. Intensivmed. Notf. Schmerzther.* **2013**, *48*, 252–257.
17. Serafini, G.; Cornara, G.; Cavalloro, F.; Mori, A.; Dore, R.; Marraro, G.; Braschi, A. Pulmonary atelectasis during paediatric anaesthesia: CT scan evaluation and effect of positive endexpiratory pressure (PEEP). *Paediatr. Anaesth.* **1999**, *9*, 225–228. [CrossRef]
18. Goldmann, K.; Roettger, C.; Wulf, H. Use of the ProSeal laryngeal mask airway for pressure-controlled ventilation with and without positive end-expiratory pressure in paediatric patients: A randomized, controlled study. *Br. J. Anaesth.* **2005**, *95*, 831–834. [CrossRef]
19. Sinha, A.; Sharma, B.; Sood, J. ProSeal laryngeal mask airway in infants and toddlers with upper respiratory tract infections: A randomized control trial of spontaneous vs pressure control ventilation. *Middle East J. Anaesthesiol.* **2009**, *20*, 437–442.
20. Lagarde, S.; Semjen, F.; Nouette-Gaulain, K.; Masson, F.; Bordes, M.; Meymat, Y.; Cros, A.M. Facemask pressure-controlled ventilation in children: What is the pressure limit? *Anesth. Analg.* **2010**, *110*, 1676–1679. [CrossRef]
21. Bouvet, L.; Albert, M.L.; Augris, C.; Boselli, E.; Ecochard, R.; Rabilloud, M.; Chassard, D.; Allaouchiche, B. Real-time detection of gastric insufflation related to facemask pressure-controlled ventilation using ultrasonography of the antrum and epigastric auscultation in nonparalyzed patients: A prospective, randomized, double-blind study. *Anesthesiology* **2014**, *120*, 326–334. [CrossRef]
22. Jagannathan, N.; Sohn, L.; Sommers, K.; Belvis, D.; Shah, R.D.; Sawardekar, A.; Eidem, J.; DaGraca, J.; Mukherji, I. A randomized comparison of the laryngeal mask airway supreme and laryngeal mask airway unique in infants and children: Does cuff pressure influence leak pressure? *Paediatr. Anaesth.* **2013**, *23*, 927–933. [CrossRef] [PubMed]
23. Wahlen, B.M.; Heinrichs, W.; Latorre, F. Gastric insufflation pressure, air leakage and respiratory mechanics in the use of the laryngeal mask airway (LMA) in children. *Paediatr. Anaesth.* **2004**, *14*, 313–317. [CrossRef] [PubMed]
24. Bernardini, A.; Natalini, G. Risk of pulmonary aspiration with laryngeal mask airway and tracheal tube: Analysis on 65 712 procedures with positive pressure ventilation. *Anaesthesia* **2009**, *64*, 1289–1294. [CrossRef] [PubMed]

Publisher's Note: MDPI stays neutral with regard to jurisdictional claims in published maps and institutional affiliations.

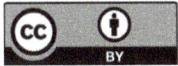

© 2020 by the authors. Licensee MDPI, Basel, Switzerland. This article is an open access article distributed under the terms and conditions of the Creative Commons Attribution (CC BY) license (http://creativecommons.org/licenses/by/4.0/).

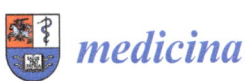

Review

Ultrasound-Guided Regional Anesthesia–Current Strategies for Enhanced Recovery after Cardiac Surgery

Cosmin Balan [1,*], Serban-Ion Bubenek-Turconi [1,2], Dana Rodica Tomescu [2,3] and Liana Valeanu [1,2]

[1] 1st Department of Cardiovascular Anesthesiology and Intensive Care, "Prof. C. C. Iliescu" Emergency Institute for Cardiovascular Diseases, 258 Fundeni Road, 022328 Bucharest, Romania; bubenek@alsys.ro (S.-I.B.-T.); liana.valeanu@yahoo.com (L.V.)

[2] Department of Anesthesiology and Intensive Care, University of Medicine and Pharmacy "Carol Davila", 8 Eroii Sanitari Blvd, 050474 Bucharest, Romania

[3] 3rd Department of Anesthesiology and Intensive Care, Fundeni Clinical Institute, 258 Fundeni Road, 022328 Bucharest, Romania; danatomescu@gmail.com

* Correspondence: cosmin13mara@yahoo.com; Tel.: +40-722751501

Abstract: With the advent of fast-track pathways after cardiac surgery, there has been a renewed interest in regional anesthesia due to its opioid-sparing effect. This paradigm shift, looking to improve resource allocation efficiency and hasten postoperative extubation and mobilization, has been pursued by nearly every specialty area in surgery. Safety concerns regarding the use of classical neuraxial techniques in anticoagulated patients have tempered the application of regional anesthesia in cardiac surgery. Recently described ultrasound-guided thoracic wall blocks have emerged as valuable alternatives to epidurals and landmark-driven paravertebral and intercostal blocks. These novel procedures enable safe, effective, opioid-free pain control. Although experience within this field is still at an early stage, available evidence indicates that their use is poised to grow and may become integral to enhanced recovery pathways for cardiac surgery patients.

Keywords: cardiac surgery; enhanced recovery; regional anesthesia; ultrasound; paravertebral blocks; fascial plane blocks; nociception level index

Citation: Balan, C.; Bubenek-Turconi, S.-I.; Tomescu, D.R.; Valeanu, L. Ultrasound-Guided Regional Anesthesia–Current Strategies for Enhanced Recovery after Cardiac Surgery. *Medicina* **2021**, *57*, 312. https://doi.org/10.3390/medicina57040312

Received: 11 February 2021
Accepted: 22 March 2021
Published: 25 March 2021

Publisher's Note: MDPI stays neutral with regard to jurisdictional claims in published maps and institutional affiliations.

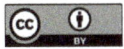

Copyright: © 2021 by the authors. Licensee MDPI, Basel, Switzerland. This article is an open access article distributed under the terms and conditions of the Creative Commons Attribution (CC BY) license (https://creativecommons.org/licenses/by/4.0/).

1. Introduction

Cardiac surgery (CS) generates a unique set of challenges compared to non-cardiac surgery. Postoperative outcomes and quality of life result from several factors, including demographic characteristics, comorbidities, type and quality of surgical intervention, the extent of the systemic inflammatory response, range of organ dysfunction and pain [1–4]. Conveniently, many of these factors are amenable to optimization. To this end, enhanced recovery after surgery (ERAS) programs have evolved and are now commanded by a multidisciplinary consensus in CS [5].

Pain management is a crucial element of cardiac ERAS. Adequate analgesia is a prerequisite to ensure patient comfort, low morbidity, early mobilization, and cost effectiveness. Postoperative pain is multifaceted and may result from various interventions, including sternotomy, thoracotomy, chest drains and leg vein harvesting. One study found that maximal pain intensity in CS was usually moderate [6], but severe acute postoperative pain was also reported elsewhere and more frequently associated with chronic post-sternotomy pain [7].

Traditionally, opioids were considered the mainstay for pain management after CS based on a predictable hemodynamic profile. Acknowledged risks associated with their use (e.g., hyperalgesia, opioid dependence, respiratory depression, nausea and vomiting, immunosuppression, ileus, delirium, prolonged postoperative recovery) fueled that which now represents a central tenet in the ERAS paradigm–multimodal analgesia (MA) [8]. MA built on drug combinations is not faultless [9]; N-methyl-D-aspartate (NMDA) antagonists may bring about sympathetic hyperactivity, central alpha-2 agonists can cause bradycardia and hypotension, and nonsteroidal anti-inflammatory agents are associated with renal dysfunction and abnormal clotting.

Regional anesthesia/analgesia (RA) represents a valid alternative for the MA repertoire. It obviates many of the drawbacks of drug-based MA strategies, albeit with its particular challenges [10]. Classical neuraxial techniques such as thoracic epidural anesthesia (TEA) and landmark-based paravertebral blocks (PVB$_{LM}$) constituted the standard regional approach to ensure chest wall pain relief before ultrasound (US) virtually revolutionized RA. Bleeding complications (e.g., spinal epidural hematoma (SEH)) were the primary concern regarding the use of TEA and PVB$_{LM}$ in CS [11]. This may explain to some extent why CS fell behind other surgical specialties regarding the large-scale implementation of ERAS programs. Since its inception, US-guided RA (USRA) has helped improve existing techniques (i.e., PVB) and favored the design of new ones. Specifically, real-time US needle-tracking is essential to perform chest wall fascial plane blocks (CWFPB) [12]. Delivery of local anesthetics (LA) between myofascial layers spares the neuraxium and blocks the nerves as they course within that tissue plane. Reasons for the growing popularity of CWFPB include (1) ease of performance; (2) excellent safety profile; (3) good efficacy in various clinical settings. The scope of this review is to address the use of RA in CS, with particular reference to the indications, techniques, and complications of currently available CWFPB (see Table A1, Appendix A).

2. Techniques

RA of the chest wall may be performed at various points along an arch coursing anteriorly from the posterior midline. With TEA as gold standard regarding the breadth of somatic and sympathetic blockade, CWFPB exhibit a variable decrement in their effect as they approach the anterior midline. Autonomic effects are retained proportionally to the extent of LA spread into the epidural space, and the area of sensory loss is inversely related to the distance between the injection spot and spine. A considerable inter-individual variation in the extent and intensity of CWFPB exists, and several reasons may represent the root cause of this: (1) existence of differential sensory blockade [13]; (2) reliance on passive LA spread to achieve analgesia; (3) redundant innervation between peripheral nerve territories, including midline overlapping [14,15].

2.1. Thoracic Epidural Anaesthesia (TEA)

The role of TEA in cardiac ERAS programs remains an intensely debated topic. TEA produces robust chest wall pain relief, yet it repeatedly failed to improve perioperative morbidity and mortality in CS populations [16]. Potential reasons include the fact that TEA benefits may have a disproportionate impact on CS pain or because TEA side effects and complications may offset its benefits. Notably, pain associated with CS is typically moderate [6], so less intense analgesia (i.e., CWFPB) might suffice. In contrast, adverse events associated with TEA may be clinically relevant (e.g., respiratory depression with epidural opioids and hypotension with epidural LA) and potentially catastrophic (e.g., SEH).

Cardiac sympatholysis was shown to benefit myocardial blood flow [17] but also blunt the heart capacity to cope with hemodynamic challenges, especially within specific subgroups such as those with established pulmonary hypertension [18].

The calculated maximum risks of SEH in CS after TEA were 1:1500 with 95% confidence and 1:1000 with 99% confidence, respectively [19]. In a recent meta-analysis of over 6000 patients, Landoni et al. estimated this risk at 1:3552 (95% CI 1:2552–1:5841) [20]. Placing the epidural one day before surgery could prevent bleeding complications, but such practice patterns would contradict the very essence of ERAS programs.

Overall, minimization of risks outweighs maximization of analgetic potential. Adequate patient selection, risk factors, and anesthesiologist's expertise must be carefully balanced before pursuing TEA or any other type of neuraxial technique. Until more evidence becomes available, the risk-benefit ratio of neuraxial analgesia remains prohibitive.

2.2. Paravertebral Blocks (PVB)

2.2.1. Mechanism and Clinical Applications

PVB involves LA injection into the thoracic paravertebral space (TPVS) to block the spinal nerve roots as they emerge from the intervertebral foramina. TPVS is a triangular-shaped space on both sides of the vertebrae bounded anterolaterally by the parietal pleura, medially by the posterolateral parts of the vertebral body and posteriorly by the superior costotransverse ligament (SCTL) (see also Figure 1). TPVS communicates laterally with the intercostal space, and medially with the epidural space. TPVS is also contiguous with its contralateral counterpart but to a much lesser extent whereas its cranial extension remains ill-defined. Caudal and rostral segmental spread of the LA drug from the injection site generates multilevel ipsilateral somatic and autonomic blockade, with epidural and intercostal LA dispersions likely contributing substantially to analgesia [21]. The clinical effect of single-level PVB_{LM} is highly variable because the LA spread is unpredictable [22]. Consequently, a multiple-injection technique was commonly considered superior to single-injection patterns [23,24]. This theory was first challenged by Renes et al. [25] and Marhofer et al. [26] who used US-guidance to perform PVB (PVB_{US}). Later, Uppal et al. [27] demonstrated that single- and multilevel PVB_{US} are equivalent regarding coverage and pain relief duration. Conveniently, the single-level PVB_{US} are markedly faster and better tolerated by patients, two prerequisites of any ERAS strategy.

Compared to PVB_{LM}, PVB_{US} are more reliable and safer [28]. Two assets, equivalent analgesia to TEA but with fewer complications [29–34] and unilateral sympathectomy, favored the resurgence of PVB_{US}. Still, the latter proves itself ineffectual in CS with sternotomy since this surgery requires bilateral nerve blockade.

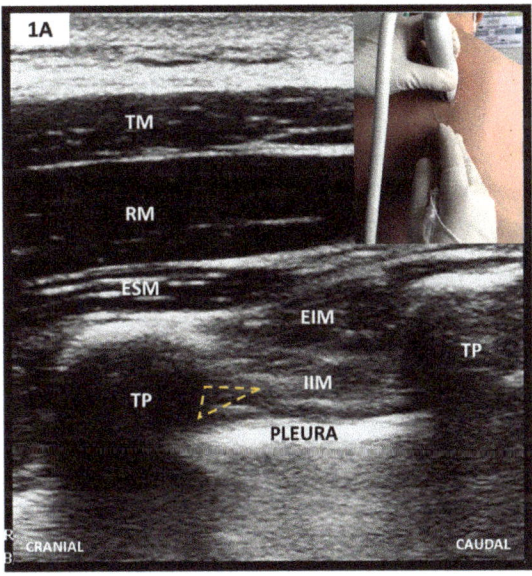

Figure 1. Cont.

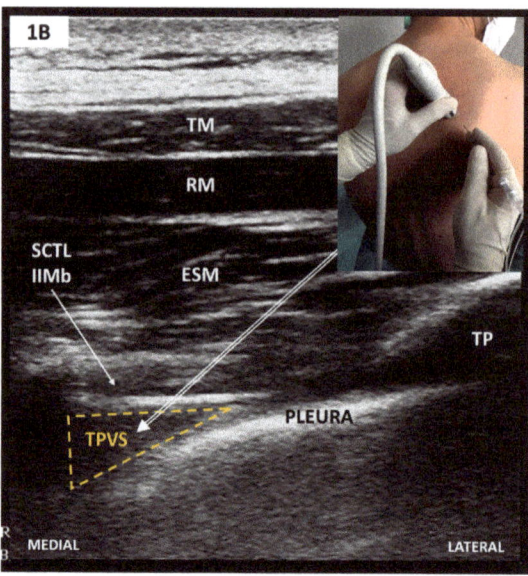

Figure 1. (**A**) Parasagittal scan of thoracic paravertebral space (TPVS); (**B**) Transverse/oblique scan of TPVS after 75-degree anti-clockwise rotation from A. The needle tip's target is TPVS, which, after probe rotation, appears enlarged and lies anteriorly to superior costotransverse ligament (SCTL)/IIMb (see text).TM, trapezius muscle; RM, rhomboid muscle; ESM, erector spinae muscle; EIM, external intercostal muscle; IIM, internal intercostal muscle; TP, transverse vertebral process; SCTL, superior costotransverse ligament; IIMb, internal intercostal membrane; TPVS, thoracic paravertebral space.

As with TEA, hemorrhagic complications represent a crucial factor to consider. In contrast to TEA, risk quantification of SEH after PVB is less evident and intensely debated. The latest American Society of Regional Anesthesia and Pain Medicine (ASRA) Practice Advisory on RA and anticoagulation maintains the same recommendations for PVB as for any other neuraxial block [11]. Equivocally, ASRA does not differentiate between PVB_{LM} and PVB_{US}, and between single-shot PVB and PVB with catheters. New data suggests that US guidance during paravertebral blockade could virtually abrogate spinal injury risk even with the large heparin dosing needed in cardiopulmonary bypass (CPB) [35]. El Shora et al. recently compared PVB_{US} with catheter to TEA to manage pain after on-pump CS [36]. Catheters were placed immediately after induction in both study groups, and LA infusion was started only postoperatively. PVB_{US} were non-inferior to TEA regarding pain relief, and bleeding complications were not reported in either group.

Future studies will have to address two aspects to maximize the benefits and minimize the potential risks associated with PVB_{US}. The first is concerned with single-shot PVB being safer than PVB with TPVS catheters because catheter misplacement, including epidurally, is still possible even with US [37,38]. The second aspect is concerned with nerve blockade timing, as suggested by Richardson et al. [39]. Compared to PVB_{US} established after surgery, preemptive PVB_{US} may be better tailored to fast-tracking as it would also mitigate the intraoperative opioid consumption.

The best strategy to implement PVB_{US} has yet to be established. Further research is needed before the routine use of paravertebral blockade in CS is either supported or refuted.

Sonoanatomy and Block Techniques (Figure 1)

PVB_{US} have superseded PVB_{LM} in every aspect. A comprehensive review described at least nine approaches, all of which share the same three sonoanatomical landmarks circumscribing TPVS—rib, pleura, and transverse process (TP) [40]. At present, formal recommendations on the best way to perform PVB_{US} do not exist. Instead, personal factors relating to skill, experience and perceived safety seem to play a decisive role. An objective comparative evaluation of currently used PVB_{US} techniques is essential to enable an informed PVB-based MA.

TPVS scanning breaks down to 4 elements: (1) plane of US beam orientation (i.e., transversal versus sagittal); (2) needling technique (i.e., out-of-plane versus in-plane); (3) direction of angulation (i.e., lateral versus medial, and caudal versus cranial respectively) and (4) safety limit for needle tip (i.e., anteriorly or posteriorly to SCTL) [40]. Choosing between these elements entails a trade-off between two goals, simplicity and accuracy. The latter is advocated in our institute, so we perform an in-plane, lateral to medial, transversal/oblique approach with a safety limit set anteriorly to SCTL (see Figure 1). Based on currently available evidence, catheters are excluded with CPB heparin dosing.

Scanning starts with the linear-array transducer placed in a parasagittal plane to identify the adjacent TP, recognizable as flat, rectangular hypoechoic structures (see also Figure 2). Anti-clockwise rotation to a transversal/oblique plane displays the TPVS. The needle is inserted in-plane, latero-medially and advanced until it reaches the wedged-shaped TPVS. Adequate LA injection pushes the parietal pleura anteriorly. Preemptive bilateral single-shot blocks are performed at the level of the fourth thoracic vertebrae. This alone may provide intraoperative analgesia long enough to sustain most types of CS.

2.3. Chest Wall Fascial Plane Blocks (CWFPB)

2.3.1. Posterior CWFPB-Erector Spinae Plane Block (ESPB) and other PVB Variants

Mechanism and Clinical Applications

Post-mortem data challenge the traditional view that TPVS is a discrete anatomical space and suggest that the SCTL is permeable to LA drugs [41]. Hence, paravertebral blockade of nerves could still be elicited by placing the needle tip outside but close enough to the TPVS.

US guidance has facilitated the emergence of several more superficial needle placement techniques, all collectively labelled as "paraspinal blocks" [42] or "PVB by proxy" [43]. These include the retrolaminar block (RLB) [44,45], midpoint transverse process to pleura block (MTPB) [41], intercostal/paraspinal block (ICPB) [46], rhomboid intercostal and subserratus block (RISS) [47], and erector spinae plane block (ESPB) [48]. Depending on their underlying pathway of LA spread, these novel blocks produce a variable combination of ipsilateral somatic and autonomic blockades, the extent of which remains open for further research. Amongst them, ESPB is the most well characterized to date.

The ESPB target for LA deposition is the plane between the erector spinae muscle (ESM) and the thoracic TP tip. Correct single-level LA injection should lift the ESM off the TP and allow the ipsilateral craniocaudal volume-dependent [49] LA spread across several contiguous dermatomes (i.e., 3 to 7 intercostal spaces) [50]. As with PVB, transforaminal, intercostal and circumferential epidural diffusions likely contribute to its mechanism of action [50,51].

Krishna et al. compared bilateral single-shot ESPB with control (i.e., general anesthesia alone) in CS with sternotomy and found reduced postoperative pain, time to extubation, time to ambulation, opioid usage and total length of intensive care unit (ICU) stay [52]. Interestingly, rescue analgesia was reported in the intervention group only ten hours after extubation compared to six hours in the control group ($p = 0.0001$). Macaire et al. used a before-and-after design to show that in open CS a preemptive strategy with bilateral ESPB catheters is associated with reduced intra- and postoperative opioid consumption. Consequently, several ERAS endpoints were favorably altered, including postoperative adverse events (hypotension, nausea/vomiting and hyperglycemia) and times to chest tube removal and first mobilization. The authors found no differences in extubation time and pain during the first mobilization. Another RCT showed comparable postoperative pain scores between bilateral continuous ESPB and TEA in 50 patients undergoing open CS [53]. Finally, Bousquet at al. endorse the association of bilateral parasternal block with bilateral ESPB [54] given that ESPB alone may sometimes fail to provide adequate parasternal analgesia [55]. This dual blockade significantly reduced the intraoperative sufentanil and postoperative morphine usage in a 20-patient cohort [54]. These four studies did not report any RA related adverse effects, but then again, neither was appropriately powered to detect them.

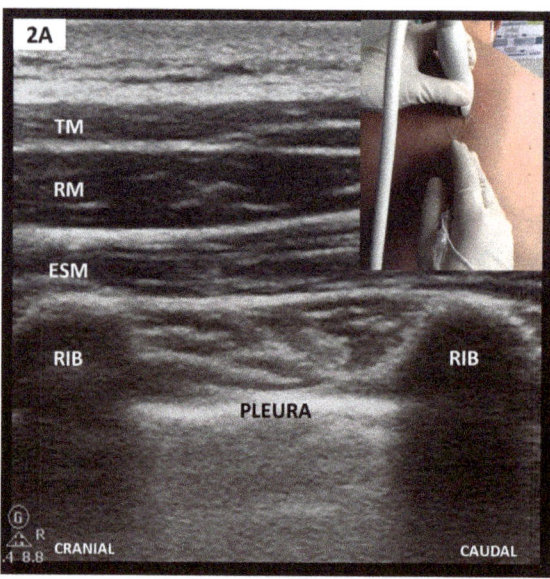

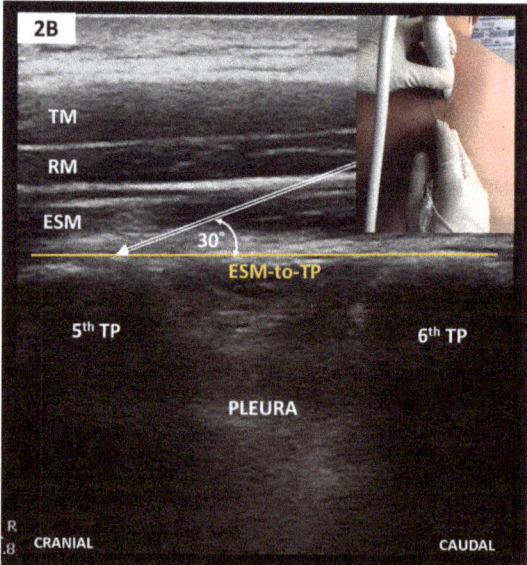

Figure 2. (**A**) Parasagittal scan—rib level; (**B**) Parasagittal scan—TP level (see text). TM, trapezius muscle; RM, rhomboid muscle; ESM, erector spinae muscle; TP, transverse vertebral process; ESM-to-TP, erector spinae muscle -to-transversus process plane.

Although promising, results from these clinical studies are not generalizable. There is a potential bias concerning the small patient populations, blinding and randomization. Further studies are mandated to fully understand the benefits and extent of incorporating ESPB into routine clinical practice.

Sonoanatomy and Block Tachnique (Figure 2)

Scanning starts with the linear-array transducer set 5–6 cm away from the dorsal midline in a parasagittal orientation. The ribs are then displayed as rounded acoustic shadows with an interceding hyperechoic pleural line (see Figure 2A). Sliding the transducer medially along the short axis allows visualization of the TP as flat, squared-off acoustic shadows (see Figure 2B). Additionally, the pleural line is more in-depth and ill-defined. A too medial position identifies the thoracic laminae as a continuous flat hyperechoic line with regularly interspersed notches representing the facet joint interfaces. Needle insertion follows an in-plane approach, either craniocaudal or vice versa, to contact the ESM-to-TP plane. Real-time imaging guarantees correct LA hydro-dissection beneath the ESM and catheter placement whenever continuous pain relief is warranted. Single-level injection ESPBs (i.e., at the 5th thoracic vertebrae), as initially described by Forero et al. [48], continue to be the norm but this view has recently been challenged by Tulgar et al. who propose a bilevel approach to ensure a more homogeneous LA spread [56].

2.3.2. Anterolateral CWFPB—Pectoral Blocks and Serratus Plane Block

Mechanism and Clinical Application

Anterolateral CWFPB provide ipsilateral somatic anesthesia of the upper anterolateral hemithorax but may spare the anterior branches of the intercostal nerves and hence do not consistently provide anesthetic coverage to the ipsilateral parasternal region [12]. This theoretically hinders their use in CS with sternotomy. Established techniques include the serratus anterior plane block (SAPB) [57] and the pectoralis block type I (PECS I) [58] and II (PECS II) [59]. Whilst PECS I and SAPB are distinct blocks, targeting two separate musculofascial planes, PECS II merely represents an attempt to achieve both PECS I and SAPB during a two-staged single needle pass (see also Figure 3).

A 40-patient RCT compared PECS II with no block as part of a postoperative MA strategy in patients undergoing CS with sternotomy. PECS group patients were extubated earlier, had lower pain scores and fewer episodes of rescue analgesia [60].

SAPB was studied in minimally invasive heart valve surgery (MIHVS) with right thoracotomy and minimally invasive direct coronary artery bypass (MIDCAB) with left thoracotomy. Berthoud et al. compared postoperative single-shot deep SAPB to continuous wound infiltration (CWI) and reported significantly lower morphine consumption, reduced length of ICU stay and improved pain control during the first 48 h following MIHVS [61]. Another group of authors compared pre-incisional single-shot and postoperative catheter-based deep SABP against parenteral morphine [62]. The intraoperative opioid usage remained unaffected, but the combined regional nerve blockade significantly spared the postoperative morphine consumption. Nevertheless, this did not change the postoperative course, that is, ICU and hospital lengths of stay and ventilator-free days. According to one study, SAPB appears well suited for MIDCAB thoracotomies [63] but remains inferior to PVB in terms of analgesic coverage and intensity [64]. Lastly, SAPB and PECS II showed an equivalent analgesic effect in an RCT conducted on pediatric patients undergoing CS with thoracotomy without CPB [65].

Anterolateral CWFPB have an excellent safety profile that will allow their ongoing integration in cardiac ERAS pathways. Their impact relies markedly on adequate timing (i.e., pre- versus postoperative blockade) and indication.

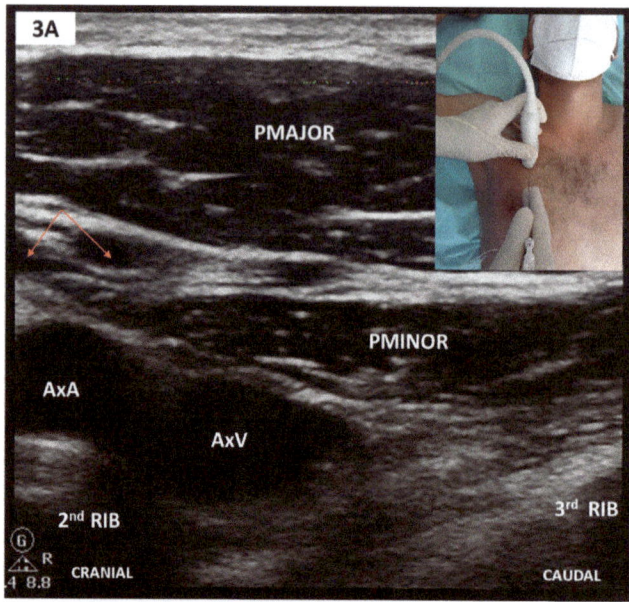
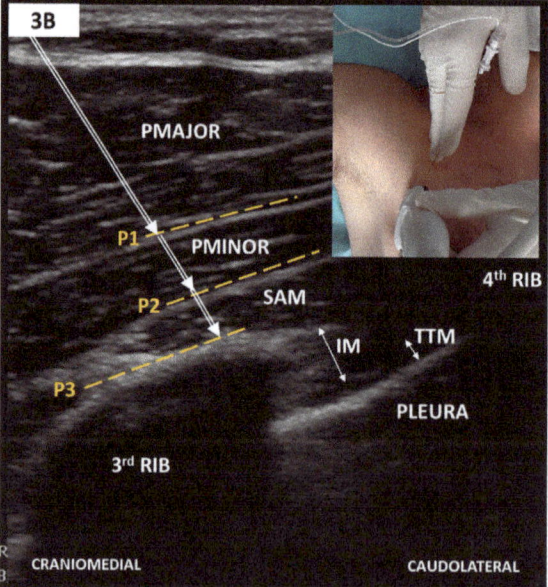

Figure 3. (**A**) Parasagittal scan along the medioclavicular line-2nd rib level; (**B**) Oblique scan after a slight medial tilt with inferolateral sliding towards the midaxillary line-4th rib level (see text). PMAJOR, pectoralis major muscle; PMINOR, pectoralis minor muscle; AxA, axillary artery; AxV, axillary vein; red arrows, thoracoacromial artery and vein; SAM, serratus anterior muscle; IM, intercostal muscle; TTM, transversus thoracic muscle; P1, PECS I plane; P2, superficial plane for SAPB/PECS II; P3, deep plane for SAPB/PECS II. To elicit an adequate SAPB coverage, P2 or P3 need to be targeted at the 4th or 5th rib level.

Sonoanatomy and Block Technique (Figure 3)

PECS I targets the lateral (C5–C7) and medial (C8–T1) pectoral nerves travelling within the fascial plane between the pectoralis minor and major muscles. SAPB targets the plane either above or below the serratus anterior muscle (SAM). Although some authors favor the latter [66], the differences between these two juxtaposed fascial planes have not yet been elucidated. SAPB blocks the lateral cutaneous branches of the intercostal branches and, when superficially performed, the long thoracic (C5–C7) and thoracodorsal nerves (C6–C8). A single needle pass may secure both blocks (i.e., PECS II) and achieve ipsilateral anesthesia of the anterolateral hemithorax and axilla. Scanning is carried out craniocaudally along the midclavicular line, sliding laterally to intersect the midaxillary line at the fourth and fifth ribs level. Needle insertion follows an in-plane, mediolateral approach (see Figure 3).

2.3.3. Anteromedial CWFPB—Parasternal Block Variants

Mechanism and Clinical Applications

These blocks complement the anterolateral CWFPB by providing anesthesia confined to the parasternal region [67]. Depending on where the anterior branches of the intercostal nerves are blocked, anteromedial CWFPB consist of two interrelated approaches: the pecto-intercostal fascial plane block (PIFB) [68] and transverse thoracic muscle plane block (TTMPB) [69]. The former is the injection of LA between the external intercostal and pectoralis major muscles. The latter targets a deeper fascial layer between the inner intercostal and transverse thoracic muscles. Some authors promote PIFB because of a potentially superior safety profile [70,71] and others inform that the transverse thoracic muscles may be too thin to identify with US [72].

Both parasternal variants have been evaluated in CS with sternotomy. Two small RCTs looked at bilateral single-shot PIFB as part of a postoperative MA regimen. Adverse effects were not recorded, and pain scores were significantly reduced in both trials [73,74]. There was a trend towards reduced cumulative opioid consumption, but this reached statistical significance in only one trial [73]. Anecdotal evidence supports the combination of PIFB with other fascial plane blocks as clinically required [75]. Furthermore, such an approach may be readily generalizable to all CWFPB and lend itself to an individualized USRA.

Preemptive single-shot bilateral TTMPB was compared with placebo in an RCT of 48 adult patients undergoing CS with median sternotomy. Several ERAS-specific outcomes were significantly improved, including first 24 h opioid requirement, rescue analgesia, pain scores, and ICU discharge time [76]. Similar findings have been reported by several pediatric RCTs in CS via midline sternotomy [77,78], with one trial using a combination of TTMPB with rectus sheath block [79].

Sonoanatomy and Block Technique (Figure 4)

The linear-array probe is placed in the parasagittal plane, 1 cm lateral from sternum's edge in the fourth or fifth intercostal space (see Figure 4). Structures to be identified include the pectoralis major muscle, intercostal muscle, thoracic transversus muscles and rib shadows with the intervening pleural line. The internal thoracic artery and vein run longitudinally and share the same plane with TTMPB (i.e., superficial to the thoracic transversus muscle). Perforating branches may cross the intercostal muscles to reach the sternum. Careful scanning in two orthogonal planes is thus mandated before needle insertion to avoid inadvertent vascular puncture. To this end, some authors recommend a transversal approach with lateral to medial needle advancement [72]. Regardless of probe orientation, one or both target planes can then be selected to deposit LA using an in-plane approach.

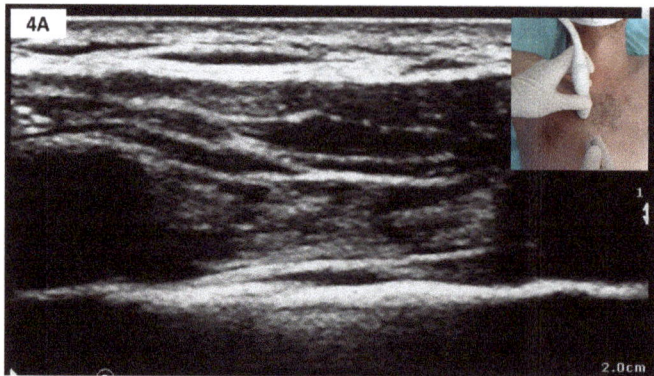
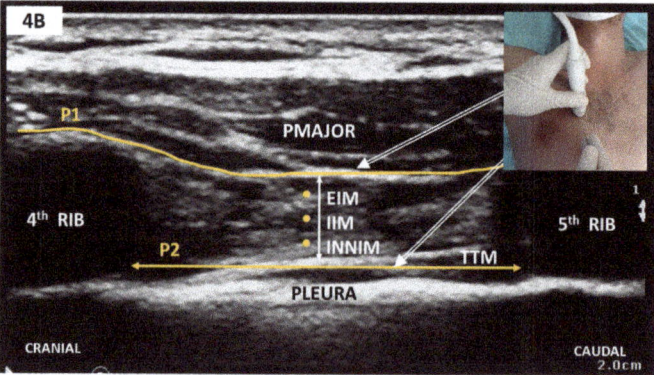

Figure 4. (**A**) Sagittal parasternal scan; (**B**) Sagittal parasternal scan with markings. Note that TTM appears as a hypoechoic band folding over the hyperechoic pleura. PMAJOR, pectoralis major muscle; EIM, external intercostal muscle; IIM, internal intercostal muscle; INNIM, innermost intercostal muscle; TTM, thoracic transversus muscle; P1, target plane for PIFB; P2, target plane for TTMPB.

3. Complications

US-assistance has dramatically increased the safety and efficiency of RA techniques resulting in improved outcomes. Reports of complications are scarce and unsystematic. Although local anesthetic systemic toxicity (LAST) is virtually a shared complication of all blocks, it may be more often reported with blocks performed in highly vascular compartments. That was the case with PVB in a case series of eight patients undergoing coronary artery bypass grafting (CABG), where potentially toxic ropivacaine concentrations were reportedly common [80]. Of note, PVB were performed using a landmark technique, and catheters were placed in all patients. Similarly, Lockwood et al. cautioned that systemic absorption after PVB_{LM} is highly probable, especially with continuous catheter infusions [81]. Such findings are compelling enough to consider, regardless of block location and technique, the following precautions: (1) do not exceed the maximum recommended LA dose (see also Table A1); (2) addition of epinephrine to delay systemic absorption; (3) be ready to monitor, recognize and treat LAST; and (4) consider US to enable precise needle advancement [82].

Sympathectomy varies in extent and intensity and is common with posterior nerve blocks, mostly bilateral PVB. Compared to PVB, posterior CWFPB seem less associated with hypotension and bradycardia [83], probably because the epidural spread is lower than initially thought [84].

Performance of PVB and CWFPB can, in theory, result in iatrogenic pneumothorax. Nevertheless, the incidence of this will remain undefined given that chest tubes are invariably present in CS with median sternotomy.

Although PVB are formally contraindicated with CPB anticoagulation regimens, the same recommendations may not apply to the more superficial CWFPB. To date, there are no reported hemorrhagic complications after any of the CWFPB, with anecdotal evidence supporting their use in contexts otherwise prohibitive for classical neuraxial techniques [85].

4. Perspective

The best way to provide RA as part of cardiac ERAS strategies has become a topic of considerable interest. Future trials are needed to compare currently available USRA techniques (e.g., PVB versus posterior and anterior CWFPB), establish the optimum time to start the nervous blockade (i.e., pre- versus postoperatively) and understand the role of various perineural adjuvants. This last issue could have momentous consequences as it may enable prolonged duration of single-injection nerve blocks and circumvent the use of catheters [86]. Catheter-free RA is faster to implement, more tolerable and perceivably safer. Furthermore, a simplified technique without additional catheter attempts may promote adherence and widespread use amongst anesthesiologists.

Monitoring regional blockade can be difficult under general anesthesia. With conscious, awake patients, preemptive blockades could be assessed by sensory testing (i.e., pinprick or cold stimulus), but this would delay the operation by at least twenty minutes. Intraoperative nociception monitors could help run an individualized and precise opioid-sparing strategy starting with induction. One trial is currently underway to evaluate the efficacy of ESPB on perioperative opioid consumption in CS with sternotomy during goal-directed anti-nociception using the Nociception Level (NOL) index (NCT04338984).

5. Conclusions

USRA favors improved outcomes coupled with an excellent safety profile and has gained considerable momentum in fast-track cardiac surgery over the last decade. Young adults (i.e., mean age 50 years) undergoing elective cardiac surgeries with relatively short aortic cross clamp times seem to derive the greatest benefits, including opioid sparing, reduced time to extubation, earlier mobilization and improved perioperative pain control. Upcoming trials are expected to provide the missing links needed to standardize the integration of RA in cardiac ERAS pathways. Until such time, USRA remains a valuable adjunct in cardiac perioperative care that calls for a personalized application encompassing both anesthesiologist's expertise and patient's characteristics.

Author Contributions: C.B. wrote the concept and first draft. All other authors reviewed and edited the manuscript. All authors have read and agreed to the published version of the manuscript.

Funding: This research received no external funding.

Institutional Review Board Statement: Not applicable.

Informed Consent Statement: Not applicable.

Data Availability Statement: Not applicable.

Acknowledgments: The authors would like to thank Adrian Wong, Department of Intensive Care Medicine and Anesthesia, King's College Hospital, Denmark Hill, London, UK for constructive criticism of the manuscript.

Conflicts of Interest: The authors declare no conflict of interest.

Appendix A

Table A1. Ultrasound-guided regional nerve blocks in cardiac surgery—technical considerations.

Block	Target Plane or Space	Target Nerve	Autonomic Blockade	Maximum Area of Sensory Loss	Surgical Approach—Best Fit	LA Volume for Single-Shot Block/Side #	Practice Patterns
PVB	TPVS	Dorsal and ventral rami of spinal nerve roots	Yes	Ipsilateral hemithorax	Sternotomy (BLB)	20–25 mL if single-level (4th TP) or 4–5 mL with multilevel strategy	• Formal contraindication with anticoagulation • Single-level equivalent to multilevel shots
ESP	ESM-to-TP	Dorsal and ventral rami of spinal nerve roots	Yes	Ipsilateral hemithorax	Sternotomy (BLB)	20 mL at the 5th TP	• Bilevel-injection to improve LA spread • Preemptive approach
PECS I	PMAJOR-to-PMINOR	Medial and lateral pectoral nerves	No	Narrow upper anterolateral chest wall	Minimally invasive thoracotomy (ULB)	15 mL at the 3rd rib	• Inadequate for sternotomy
PECS II	PMAJOR-to-PMINOR (1) and SUPRA- or SUB-SAM (2)	PECS I, LTN and TDN	No	Wide upper anterolateral chest wall, including axilla	Minimally invasive thoracotomy (ULB)	30 mL at the 3rd rib	• Inadequate for sternotomy • Perform (1) after (2) with a single-pass approach
SAPB	SUPRA- or SUB-SAM	Lateral branches of ICN, including LTN and TDN with superficial SABP	No	Lateral chest wall	Minimally invasive thoracotomy (ULB)	30–40 mL at the 4th–5th rib	• Inadequate for sternotomy • Anterior spread with deep SAPB; posterior spread with superficial SAPB
PIFB	PMAJOR-to-EIM	Anterior branches of ICN	No	Parasternal	Sternotomy (BLB)	20 mL at the 4th rib	• Combined
TTMPB	INNIM-to-TTM	Anterior branches of ICN	No	Parasternal	Sternotomy (BLB)	20 mL at the 4th rib	• Combined

\#—Single-shot blocks refer to one time LA injection without catheter placement. Depending on block technique, either single-level or multilevel LA deposition may be performed. Commonly used LA drugs are ropivacaine and bupivacaine with concentrations ranging from 0.25% to 0.5%. Maximum recommended doses are 2 mg/kg for bupivacaine and 3 mg/kg for ropivacaine, respectively [87]. PVB, paravertebral block; ESPB, erector spinae plane block; PECS I and II, pectoralis nerve blocks I and II; SAPB, serratus anterior plane block; PIFB, pecto-intercostal fascial plane block; TTMB, thoracic transversus plane block; TPVS, thoracic paravertebral space; ESM, erector spinae muscle; TP, thoracic transversus process; PMAJOR, pectoralis major muscle; PMINOR, pectoralis minor muscle; SAM, serratus anterior muscle; EIM, external intercostal muscle; INNIM, innermost intercostal muscle; TTM, thoracic transversus muscle; LTN, long thoracic nerve; TDN, thoracodorsal nerve; ICN, intercostal nerve; ULB, unilateral block; BLB, bilateral block.

References

1. Roques, F.; Nashef, S.A.M.; Michel, P.; Gauducheau, E.; De Vincentiis, C.; Baudet, E.; Cortina, J.; David, M.; Faichney, A.; Gavrielle, F.; et al. Risk factors and outcome in European cardiac surgery: Analysis of the EuroSCORE multinational database of 19030 patients. *Eur. J. Cardio-Thoracic. Surg.* **1999**, *15*, 816–823. [CrossRef]
2. Wahba, A.; Milojevic, M.; Boer, C.; De Somer, F.M.; Gudbjartsson, T.; van den Goor, J.; Jones, T.J.; Lomivorotov, V.; Merkle, F.; Ranucci, M.; et al. 2019 EACTS/EACTA/EBCP guidelines on cardiopulmonary bypass in adult cardiac surgery. *Br. J. Anaesth.* **2019**, *123*, 713–757. [CrossRef]
3. Ranucci, M. Anaesthesia and cardiopulmonary bypass aspects of fast track. *Eur. Hear. J. Suppl.* **2017**, *19*, A15–A17. [CrossRef]
4. Gerstein, N.S.; Petersen, T.R.; Ramakrishna, H. Evaluating the Cardiac Anesthesiologist's Role in Surgical Outcomes—A Reappraisal Based on Recent Evidence. *J. Cardiothorac. Vasc. Anesth.* **2017**, *31*, 283–290. [CrossRef]
5. Engelman, D.T.; Ali, W.B.; Williams, J.B.; Perrault, L.P.; Reddy, V.S.; Arora, R.C.; Roselli, E.E.; Khoynezhad, A.; Gerdisch, M.; Levy, J.H.; et al. Guidelines for Perioperative Care in Cardiac Surgery: Enhanced Recovery After Surgery Society Recommendations. *JAMA Surg.* **2019**, *154*, 755–766. [CrossRef]
6. Mueller, X.M.; Tinguely, F.; Tevaearai, H.T.; Revelly, J.P.; Chioléro, R.; von Segesser, L.K. Pain location, distribution, and intensity after cardiac surgery. *Chest* **2000**, *118*, 391–396. [CrossRef]
7. Lahtinen, P.; Kokki, H.; Hynynen, M. Pain after cardiac surgery: A prospective cohort study of 1-year incidence and intensity. *Anesthesiology* **2006**, *105*, 794–800. [CrossRef]
8. Ochroch, J.; Usman, A.; Kiefer, J.; Pulton, D.; Shah, R.; Grosh, T.; Patel, S.; Vernick, W.; Gutsche, J.T.; Raiten, J. Reducing Opioid Use in Patients Undergoing Cardiac Surgery—Preoperative, Intraoperative, and Critical Care Strategies. *J. Cardiothorac. Vasc. Anesth.* **2020**. [CrossRef]
9. Shanthanna, H.; Ladha, K.S.; Kehlet, H.; Joshi, G.P. Perioperative Opioid Administration: A Critical Review of Opioid-free versus Opioid-sparing Approaches. *Anesthesiology* **2020**. [CrossRef]
10. Mittnacht, A.J.; Shariat, A.; Weiner, M.M.; Malhotra, A.; Miller, M.A.; Mahajan, A.; Bhatt, H.V. Regional Techniques for Cardiac and Cardiac-Related Procedures. *J. Cardiothorac. Vasc. Anesth.* **2019**, *33*, 532–546. [CrossRef] [PubMed]
11. Horlocker, T.T.; Vandermeuelen, E.; Kopp, S.L.; Gogarten, W.; Leffert, L.R.; Benzon, H.T. Regional Anesthesia in the Patient Receiving Antithrombotic or Thrombolytic Therapy: American Society of Regional Anesthesia and Pain Medicine Evidence-Based Guidelines (Fourth Edition). *Reg. Anesth. Pain Med.* **2018**, *43*, 263–309. Available online: http://rapm.bmj.com/content/43/3/263.abstract (accessed on 20 January 2021). [CrossRef]
12. Kelava, M.; Alfirevic, A.; Bustamante, S.; Hargrave, J.; Marciniak, D. Regional Anesthesia in Cardiac Surgery: An Overview of Fascial Plane Chest Wall Blocks. *Anesth Analg* **2020**, *131*, 127–135. Available online: https://journals.lww.com/anesthesia-analgesia/Fulltext/2020/07000/Regional_Anesthesia_in_Cardiac_Surgery__An.23.aspx (accessed on 20 January 2021). [CrossRef]
13. Raymond, S.A.; Gissen, A.J. Mechanisms of Differential Nerve Block BT. In *Local Anesthetics*; Strichartz, G.R., Ed.; Springer: Berlin/Heidelberg, Germany, 1987; pp. 95–164. [CrossRef]
14. Capek, S.; Tubbs, R.S.; Spinner, R.J. Do cutaneous nerves cross the midline? *Clin. Anat.* **2015**, *28*, 96–100. [CrossRef]
15. Ladak, A.; Tubbs, R.S.; Spinner, R.J. Mapping sensory nerve communications between peripheral nerve territories. *Clin. Anat.* **2014**, *27*, 681–690. [CrossRef]
16. Guay, J.; Kopp, S. Epidural analgesia for adults undergoing cardiac surgery with or without cardiopulmonary bypass. *Cochrane Database Syst. Rev.* **2019**, *3*, CD006715. [CrossRef]
17. Bulte, C.S.; Boer, C.; Hartemink, K.J.; Kamp, O.; Heymans, M.W.; Loer, S.A.; de Marchi, S.F.; Vogel, R.; Bouwman, R.A. Myocardial Microvascular Responsiveness During Acute Cardiac Sympathectomy Induced by Thoracic Epidural Anesthesia. *J. Cardiothorac. Vasc. Anesth.* **2017**, *31*, 134–141. [CrossRef] [PubMed]
18. Wink, J.; Veering, B.T.; Aarts, L.P.H.J.; Wouters, P.F. Effects of Thoracic Epidural Anesthesia on Neuronal Cardiac Regulation and Cardiac Function. *Anesthesiology* **2019**, *130*, 472–491. [CrossRef]
19. Ho, A.M.; Chung, D.C.; Joynt, G.M. Neuraxial blockade and hematoma in cardiac surgery: Estimating the risk of a rare adverse event that has not (yet) occurred. *Chest* **2000**, *117*, 551–555. [CrossRef]
20. Landoni, G.; Isella, F.; Greco, M.; Zangrillo, A.; Royse, C.F. Benefits and risks of epidural analgesia in cardiac surgery. *BJA Br. J. Anaesth.* **2015**, *115*, 25–32. [CrossRef]
21. Karmakar, M.K. Thoracic Paravertebral Block. *Anesthesiology* **2001**, *95*, 771–780. [CrossRef]
22. Cowie, B.; McGlade, D.; Ivanusic, J.; Barrington, M.J. Ultrasound-guided thoracic paravertebral blockade: A cadaveric study. *Anesth. Analg.* **2010**, *110*, 1735–1739. [CrossRef] [PubMed]
23. Naja, Z.M.; El-Rajab, M.; Al-Tannir, M.A.; Ziade, F.M.; Tayara, K.; Younes, F.; Lönnqvist, P.A. Thoracic paravertebral block: Influence of the number of injections. *Reg. Anesth. Pain Med.* **2006**, *31*, 196–201. [CrossRef]
24. Kotzé, A.; Scally, A.; Howell, S. Efficacy and safety of different techniques of paravertebral block for analgesia after thoracotomy: A systematic review and metaregression. *Br. J. Anaesth.* **2009**, *103*, 626–636. [CrossRef]
25. Renes, S.H.; Bruhn, J.; Gielen, M.J.; Scheffer, G.J.; van Geffen, G.J. In-plane ultrasound-guided thoracic paravertebral block: A preliminary report of 36 cases with radiologic confirmation of catheter position. *Reg. Anesth. Pain Med.* **2010**, *35*, 212–216. [CrossRef]

26. Marhofer, D.; Marhofer, P.; Kettner, S.C.; Fleischmann, E.; Prayer, D.; Schernthaner, M.; Lackner, E.; Willschke, H.; Schwetz, P.; Zeitlinger, M. Magnetic resonance imaging analysis of the spread of local anesthetic solution after ultrasound-guided lateral thoracic paravertebral blockade: A volunteer study. *Anesthesiology* **2013**, *118*, 1106–1112. [CrossRef] [PubMed]
27. Uppal, V.; Sondekoppam, R.V.; Sodhi, P.; Johnston, D.; Ganapathy, S. Single-Injection Versus Multiple-Injection Technique of Ultrasound-Guided Paravertebral Blocks: A Randomized Controlled Study Comparing Dermatomal Spread. *Reg. Anesth. Pain Med.* **2017**, *42*, 575–581. [CrossRef]
28. Vogt, A. Review about ultrasounds in paravertebral blocks. *Eur. J. Pain Suppl.* **2011**, *5*, 489–494. Available online: http://www.sciencedirect.com/science/article/pii/S1754320711000460 (accessed on 24 January 2021). [CrossRef]
29. D'Ercole, F.; Arora, H.; Kumar, P.A. Paravertebral Block for Thoracic Surgery. *J. Cardiothorac. Vasc. Anesth.* **2018**, *32*, 915–927. [CrossRef]
30. Baidya, D.K.; Khanna, P.; Maitra, S. Analgesic efficacy and safety of thoracic paravertebral and epidural analgesia for thoracic surgery: A systematic review and meta-analysis. *Interact. Cardiovasc. Thorac. Surg.* **2014**, *18*, 626–635. [CrossRef] [PubMed]
31. Yeung, J.H.Y.; Gates, S.; Naidu, B.V.; Wilson, M.J.A.; Gao Smith, F. Paravertebral block versus thoracic epidural for patients undergoing thoracotomy. *Cochrane Database Syst. Rev.* **2016**, *2*, CD009121. [CrossRef]
32. Scarci, M.; Joshi, A.; Attia, R. In patients undergoing thoracic surgery is paravertebral block as effective as epidural analgesia for pain management? *Interact. Cardiovasc. Thorac. Surg.* **2010**, *10*, 92–96. [CrossRef] [PubMed]
33. Davies, R.G.; Myles, P.S.; Graham, J.M. A comparison of the analgesic efficacy and side-effects of paravertebral vs epidural blockade for thoracotomy—A systematic review and meta-analysis of randomized trials. *Br. J. Anaesth.* **2006**, *96*, 418–426. [CrossRef]
34. Scarfe, A.J.; Schuhmann-Hingel, S.; Duncan, J.K.; Ma, N.; Atukorale, Y.N.; Cameron, A.L. Continuous paravertebral block for post-cardiothoracic surgery analgesia: A systematic review and meta-analysis. *Eur. J. Cardio-Thoracic. Surg. Off. J. Eur. Assoc. Cardio-Thoracic. Surg.* **2016**, *50*, 1010–1018. [CrossRef] [PubMed]
35. Okitsu, K.; Iritakenishi, T.; Iwasaki, M.; Imada, T.; Fujino, Y. Risk of Hematoma in Patients With a Bleeding Risk Undergoing Cardiovascular Surgery With a Paravertebral Catheter. *J. Cardiothorac. Vasc. Anesth.* **2017**, *31*, 453–457. [CrossRef]
36. El Shora, H.A.; El Beleehy, A.A.; Abdelwahab, A.A.; Ali, G.A.; Omran, T.E.; Hassan, E.A.; Arafat, A.A. Bilateral Paravertebral Block versus Thoracic Epidural Analgesia for Pain Control Post-Cardiac Surgery: A Randomized Controlled Trial. *Thorac. Cardiovasc. Surg.* **2020**, *68*, 410–416. [CrossRef]
37. Luyet, C.; Herrmann, G.; Ross, S.; Vogt, A.; Greif, R.; Moriggl, B.; Eichenberger, U. Ultrasound-guided thoracic paravertebral puncture and placement of catheters in human cadavers: Where do catheters go? *Br. J. Anaesth.* **2011**, *106*, 246–254. [CrossRef]
38. Luyet, C.; Eichenberger, U.; Greif, R.; Vogt, A.; Szücs Farkas, Z.; Moriggl, B. Ultrasound-guided paravertebral puncture and placement of catheters in human cadavers: An imaging study. *Br. J. Anaesth.* **2009**, *102*, 534–539. [CrossRef] [PubMed]
39. Richardson, J.; Sabanathan, S.; Jones, J.; Shah, R.D.; Cheema, S.; Mearns, A.J. A prospective, randomized comparison of preoperative and continuous balanced epidural or paravertebral bupivacaine on post-thoracotomy pain, pulmonary function and stress responses. *Br. J. Anaesth.* **1999**, *83*, 387–392. [CrossRef] [PubMed]
40. Krediet, A.C.; Moayeri, N.; van Geffen, G.J.; Bruhn, J.; Renes, S.; Bigeleisen, P.E.; Groen, G.J. Different Approaches to Ultrasound-guided Thoracic Paravertebral Block: An Illustrated Review. *Anesthesiology* **2015**, *123*, 459–474. [CrossRef] [PubMed]
41. Costache, I.; De Neumann, L.; Ramnanan, C.J.; Goodwin, S.L.; Pawa, A.; Abdallah, F.W.; McCartney, C.J.L. The mid-point transverse process to pleura (MTP) block: A new end-point for thoracic paravertebral block. *Anaesthesia* **2017**, *72*, 1230–1236. [CrossRef] [PubMed]
42. Wild, K.; Chin, K.J. Regional Techniques for Thoracic Wall Surgery. *Curr. Anesthesiol. Rep.* **2017**, *7*, 212–219. [CrossRef]
43. Costache, I.; Pawa, A.; Abdallah, F.W. Paravertebral by proxy—Time to redefine the paravertebral block. *Anaesthesia* **2018**, *73*, 1185–1188. [CrossRef]
44. Voscopoulos, C.; Palaniappan, D.; Zeballos, J.; Ko, H.; Janfaza, D.; Vlassakov, K. The ultrasound-guided retrolaminar block. *Can. J. Anaesth.* **2013**, *60*, 888–895. [CrossRef]
45. Murouchi, T.; Yamakage, M. Retrolaminar block: Analgesic efficacy and safety evaluation. *J. Anesth.* **2016**, *30*, 1003–1007. [CrossRef]
46. Roué, C.; Wallaert, M.; Kacha, M.; Havet, E. Intercostal/paraspinal nerve block for thoracic surgery. *Anaesthesia* **2016**, *71*, 112–113. [CrossRef]
47. Elsharkawy, H.; Maniker, R.; Bolash, R.; Kalasbail, P.; Drake, R.L.; Elkassabany, N. Rhomboid Intercostal and Subserratus Plane Block: A Cadaveric and Clinical Evaluation. *Reg. Anesth. Pain Med.* **2018**, *43*, 745–751. [CrossRef]
48. Forero, M.; Adhikary, S.D.; Lopez, H.; Tsui, C.; Chin, K.J. The Erector Spinae Plane Block: A Novel Analgesic Technique in Thoracic Neuropathic Pain. *Reg. Anesth. Pain Med.* **2016**, *41*, 621–627. [CrossRef] [PubMed]
49. Choi, Y.J.; Kwon, H.J.; O, J.; Cho, T.H.; Won, J.Y.; Yang, H.M.; Kim, S.H. Influence of injectate volume on paravertebral spread in erector spinae plane block: An endoscopic and anatomical evaluation. *PLoS ONE* **2019**, *14*, e0224487. Available online: https://pubmed.ncbi.nlm.nih.gov/31658293 (accessed on 4 February 2021). [CrossRef] [PubMed]
50. Vidal, E.; Giménez, H.; Forero, M.; Fajardo, M. Erector spinae plane block: A cadaver study to determine its mechanism of action. *Rev. Esp. Anestesiol. Reanim.* **2018**, *65*, 514–519. [CrossRef]
51. Schwartzmann, A.; Peng, P.; Maciel, M.A.; Forero, M. Mechanism of the erector spinae plane block: Insights from a magnetic resonance imaging study. *Can. J. Anaesth.* **2018**, *65*, 1165–1166. [CrossRef]

52. Krishna, S.N.; Chauhan, S.; Bhoi, D.; Kaushal, B.; Hasija, S.; Sangdup, T.; Bisoi, A.K. Bilateral Erector Spinae Plane Block for Acute Post-Surgical Pain in Adult Cardiac Surgical Patients: A Randomized Controlled Trial. *J. Cardiothorac. Vasc. Anesth.* **2019**, *33*, 368–375. [CrossRef]
53. Nagaraja, P.S.; Ragavendran, S.; Singh, N.G.; Asai, O.; Bhavya, G.; Manjunath, N.; Rajesh, K. Comparison of continuous thoracic epidural analgesia with bilateral erector spinae plane block for perioperative pain management in cardiac surgery. *Ann. Card. Anaesth.* **2018**, *21*, 323–327.
54. Bousquet, P.; Labaste, F.; Gobin, J.; Marcheix, B.; Minville, V. Bilateral Parasternal Block and Bilateral Erector Spinae Plane Block Reduce Opioid Consumption in During Cardiac Surgery. *J. Cardiothorac. Vasc. Anesth.* **2021**. [CrossRef]
55. Taketa, Y.; Irisawa, Y.; Fujitani, T. Ultrasound-guided erector spinae plane block elicits sensory loss around the lateral, but not the parasternal, portion of the thorax. *J. Clin. Anesth.* **2018**, *47*, 84–85. [CrossRef] [PubMed]
56. Tulgar, S.; Selvi, O.; Ozer, Z. Clinical experience of ultrasound-guided single and bi-level erector spinae plane block for postoperative analgesia in patients undergoing thoracotomy. *J. Clin. Anesth.* **2018**, *50*, 22–23. [CrossRef] [PubMed]
57. Blanco, R.; Parras, T.; McDonnell, J.G.; Prats-Galino, A. Serratus plane block: A novel ultrasound-guided thoracic wall nerve block. *Anaesthesia* **2013**, *68*, 1107–1113. [CrossRef] [PubMed]
58. Blanco, R. The "pecs block": A novel technique for providing analgesia after breast surgery. *Anaesthesia* **2011**, *66*, 847–848. [CrossRef]
59. Blanco, R.; Fajardo, M.; Parras Maldonado, T. Ultrasound description of Pecs II (modified Pecs I): A novel approach to breast surgery. *Rev. Esp. Anestesiol. Reanim.* **2012**, *59*, 470–475. [CrossRef]
60. Kumar, K.N.; Kalyane, R.N.; Singh, N.G.; Nagaraja, P.S.; Krishna, M.; Babu, B.; Varadaraju, R.; Sathish, N.; Manjunatha, N. Efficacy of bilateral pectoralis nerve block for ultrafast tracking and postoperative pain management in cardiac surgery. *Ann. Card. Anaesth.* **2018**, *21*, 333–338.
61. Berthoud, V.; Ellouze, O.; Nguyen, M.; Konstantinou, M.; Aho, S.; Malapert, G.; Girard, C.; Guinot, P.G.; Bouchot, O.; Bouhemad, B. Serratus anterior plane block for minimal invasive heart surgery. *BMC Anesthesiol.* **2018**, *18*, 144. [CrossRef]
62. Toscano, A.; Capuano, P.; Costamagna, A.; Burzio, C.; Ellena, M.; Scala, V.; Pasero, D.; Rinaldi, M.; Brazzi, L. The Serratus Anterior Plane Study: Continuous Deep Serratus Anterior Plane Block for Mitral Valve Surgery Performed in Right Minithoracotomy. *J. Cardiothorac. Vasc. Anesth.* **2020**, *34*, 2975–2982. [CrossRef] [PubMed]
63. Gautam, S.; Pande, S.; Agarwal, A.; Agarwal, S.K.; Rastogi, A.; Shamshery, C.; Singh, A. Evaluation of Serratus Anterior Plane Block for Pain Relief in Patients Undergoing MIDCAB Surgery. *Innovations* **2020**, *15*, 148–154. [CrossRef]
64. Moll, V.; Maffeo, C.; Mitchell, M.; Ward, C.T.; Groff, R.F.; Lee, S.C.; Halkos, M.E.; Jabaley, C.S.; O'Reilly-Shah, V.N. Association of Serratus Anterior Plane Block for Minimally Invasive Direct Coronary Artery Bypass Surgery With Higher Opioid Consumption: A Retrospective Observational Study. *J. Cardiothorac. Vasc. Anesth.* **2018**, *32*, 2570–2577. [CrossRef]
65. Kaushal, B.; Chauhan, S.; Saini, K.; Bhoi, D.; Bisoi, A.K.; Sangdup, T.; Khan, M.A. Comparison of the Efficacy of Ultrasound-Guided Serratus Anterior Plane Block, Pectoral Nerves II Block, and Intercostal Nerve Block for the Management of Postoperative Thoracotomy Pain After Pediatric Cardiac Surgery. *J. Cardiothorac. Vasc. Anesth.* **2019**, *33*, 418–425. [CrossRef]
66. Pérez, M.F.; Duany, O.; de la Torre, P.A. Redefining PECS Blocks for Postmastectomy Analgesia. *Reg. Anesth. Pain Med.* **2015**, *40*, 729–730. [CrossRef] [PubMed]
67. Ueshima, H.; Otake, H. Addition of transversus thoracic muscle plane block to pectoral nerves block provides more effective perioperative pain relief than pectoral nerves block alone for breast cancer surgery. *BJA Br. J. Anaesth.* **2017**, *118*, 439–443. [CrossRef]
68. De la Torre, P.A.; García, P.D.; Alvarez, S.L.; Miguel, F.J.G.; Pérez, M.F. A novel ultrasound-guided block: A promising alternative for breast analgesia. *Aesthetic. Surg. J.* **2014**, *34*, 198–200. [CrossRef]
69. Ueshima, H.; Kitamura, A. Blocking of Multiple Anterior Branches of Intercostal Nerves (Th2-6) Using a Transversus Thoracic Muscle Plane Block. *Reg. Anesth. Pain Med.* **2015**, *40*, 388. [CrossRef] [PubMed]
70. Scimia, P.; Fusco, P.; Tedesco, M.; Sepolvere, G. Bilateral ultrasound-guided parasternal block for postoperative analgesia in cardiac surgery: Could it be the safest strategy? *Reg. Anesth. Pain Med.* **2020**. Available online: http://rapm.bmj.com/content/early/2020/01/19/rapm-2019-100872.abstract (accessed on 20 January 2021). [CrossRef]
71. Del Buono, R.; Costa, F.; Agrò, F.E. Parasternal, Pecto-intercostal, Pecs, and Transverse Thoracic Muscle Plane Blocks: A Rose by Any Other Name Would Smell as Sweet. *Reg. Anesth. Pain Med.* **2016**, *41*, 791–792. Available online: http://rapm.bmj.com/content/41/6/791.abstract (accessed on 1 November 2020). [CrossRef]
72. Murata, H.; Hida, K.; Hara, T. Transverse Thoracic Muscle Plane Block: Tricks and Tips to Accomplish the Block. *Reg. Anesth. Pain Med.* **2016**, *41*, 411–412. Available online: http://rapm.bmj.com/content/41/3/411.2.abstract (accessed on 1 November 2020). [CrossRef] [PubMed]
73. Kumar, A.K.; Chauhan, S.; Bhoi, D.; Kaushal, B. Pectointercostal Fascial Block (PIFB) as a Novel Technique for Postoperative Pain Management in Patients Undergoing Cardiac Surgery. *J. Cardiothorac. Vasc. Anesth.* **2021**, *35*, 116–122. [CrossRef] [PubMed]
74. Khera, T.; Murugappan, K.R.; Leibowitz, A.; Bareli, N.; Shankar, P.; Gilleland, S.; Wilson, K.; Oren-Grinberg, A.; Novack, V.; Venkatachalam, S.; et al. Ultrasound-Guided Pecto-Intercostal Fascial Block for Postoperative Pain Management in Cardiac Surgery: A Prospective, Randomized, Placebo-Controlled Trial. *J. Cardiothorac. Vasc. Anesth.* **2021**, *35*, 896–903. [CrossRef]
75. Jones, J.; Murin, P.J.; Tsui, J.H. Combined Pectoral-Intercostal Fascial Plane and Rectus Sheath Blocks for Opioid-Sparing Pain Control After Extended Sternotomy for Traumatic Nail Gun Injury. *J. Cardiothorac. Vasc. Anesth.* **2021**. [CrossRef]

76. Aydin, M.E.; Ahiskalioglu, A.; Ates, I.; Tor, I.H.; Borulu, F.; Erguney, O.D.; Celik, M.; Dogan, N. Efficacy of Ultrasound-Guided Transversus Thoracic Muscle Plane Block on Postoperative Opioid Consumption After Cardiac Surgery: A Prospective, Randomized, Double-Blind Study. *J. Cardiothorac. Vasc. Anesth.* **2020**, *34*, 2996–3003. [CrossRef] [PubMed]
77. Abdelbaser, I.I.; Mageed, N.A. Analgesic efficacy of ultrasound guided bilateral transversus thoracis muscle plane block in pediatric cardiac surgery: A randomized, double-blind, controlled study. *J. Clin. Anesth.* **2020**, *67*, 110002. [CrossRef]
78. Zhang, Y.; Chen, S.; Gong, H.; Zhan, B. Efficacy of Bilateral Transversus Thoracis Muscle Plane Block in Pediatric Patients Undergoing Open Cardiac Surgery. *J. Cardiothorac. Vasc. Anesth.* **2020**, *34*, 2430–2434. [CrossRef] [PubMed]
79. Yamamoto, T.; Seino, Y.; Matsuda, K.; Imai, H.; Bamba, K.; Sugimoto, A.; Shiraishi, S.; Schindler, E. Preoperative Implementation of Transverse Thoracic Muscle Plane Block and Rectus Sheath Block Combination for Pediatric Cardiac Surgery. *J. cardioThorac. Vasc. Anesth.* **2020**, *34*, 3367–3372. Available online: https://www.sciencedirect.com/science/article/pii/S1053077020307126 (accessed on 1 November 2020). [CrossRef]
80. Ho, A.H.; Karmakar, M.K.; Ng, S.K.; Wan, S.; Ng, C.S.H.; Wong, R.H.L.; Chan, S.K.C.; Joynt, G.M. Local anaesthetic toxicity after bilateral thoracic paravertebral block in patients undergoing coronary artery bypass surgery. *Anaesth. Intensive Care* **2016**, *44*, 615–619. [CrossRef]
81. Lockwood, G.G.; Cabreros, L.; Banach, D.; Punjabi, P.P. Continuous bilateral thoracic paravertebral blockade for analgesia after cardiac surgery: A randomised, controlled trial. *Perfusion* **2017**, *32*, 591–597. [CrossRef]
82. Chin, K.J. Thoracic wall blocks: From paravertebral to retrolaminar to serratus to erector spinae and back again—A review of evidence. *Best Pract. Res. Clin. Anaesthesiol.* **2019**, *33*, 67–77. [CrossRef] [PubMed]
83. Fang, B.; Wang, Z.; Huang, X. Ultrasound-guided preoperative single-dose erector spinae plane block provides comparable analgesia to thoracic paravertebral block following thoracotomy: A single center randomized controlled double-blind study. *Ann. Transl. Med.* **2019**, *7*, 174. [CrossRef]
84. Chin, K.J.; El-Boghdadly, K. Mechanisms of action of the erector spinae plane (ESP) block: A narrative review. *Can. J. Anesth. Can. D'anesthésie* **2021**. [CrossRef] [PubMed]
85. De Cassai, A.; Ieppariello, G.; Ori, C. Erector spinae plane block and dual antiplatelet therapy. *Minerva. Anestesiol.* **2018**, *84*, 1230–1231. [CrossRef]
86. Gao, Z.; Xiao, Y.; Wang, Q.; Li, Y. Comparison of dexmedetomidine and dexamethasone as adjuvant for ropivacaine in ultrasound-guided erector spinae plane block for video-assisted thoracoscopic lobectomy surgery: A randomized, double-blind, placebo-controlled trial. *Ann. Transl. Med.* **2019**, *7*, 668. [CrossRef] [PubMed]
87. Josh Luftig, P.A.; Mantuani, D.; Herring, A.A.; Dixon, B.; Clattenburg, E.; Nagdev, A. The authors reply to the optimal dose and volume of local anesthetic for erector spinae plane blockade for posterior rib fractures. *Am. J. Emerg. Med.* **2018**, *36*, 1103–1104. [CrossRef]

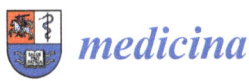

Review

Multiparametric Monitoring of Hypnosis and Nociception-Antinociception Balance during General Anesthesia—A New Era in Patient Safety Standards and Healthcare Management

Alexandru Florin Rogobete [1,2,3], Ovidiu Horea Bedreag [1,2,3,†], Marius Papurica [1,2,3,†], Sonia Elena Popovici [1,2,3,*], Lavinia Melania Bratu [1,*], Andreea Rata [4,5], Claudiu Rafael Barsac [1,2,3], Andra Maghiar [1,2], Dragos Nicolae Garofil [6], Mihai Negrea [7], Laura Bostangiu Petcu [8], Daiana Toma [2,3], Corina Maria Dumbuleu [2,3], Samir Rimawi [3] and Dorel Sandesc [1,2,3,†]

1. Faculty of Medicine, "Victor Babes" University of Medicine and Pharmacy, 300041 Timisoara, Romania; alexandru.rogobete@umft.ro (A.F.R.); bedreag.ovidiu@umft.ro (O.H.B.); marius.papurica@gmail.com (M.P.); claudiu_barsac@yahoo.com (C.R.B.); andramaghiar@yahoo.com (A.M.); dsandesc@yahoo.com (D.S.)
2. Anaesthesia and Intensive Care Research Center, "Victor Babes" University of Medicine and Pharmacy, 300041 Timisoara, Romania; daiana.toma@yahoo.com (D.T.); corina.maria.d@gmail.com (C.M.D.)
3. Clinic of Anaesthesia and Intensive Care, Emergency County Hospital "Pius Brinzeu", 300723 Timisoara, Romania; rimawi.samir@gmail.com
4. Department of Vascular Surgery, "Victor Babes" University of Medicine and Pharmacy, 300041 Timisoara, Romania; rataandreealuciana@gmail.com
5. Clinic of Vascular Surgery, Emergency County Hospital "Pius Brinzeu", 300723 Timisoara, Romania
6. Faculty of Medicine, "Carol Davila" University of Medicine and Pharmacy, 020021 Bucharest, Romania; dragosgarofil@gmail.com
7. Faculty of Political, Administrative and Communication Sciences, Babes-Bolyai University, 400376 Cluj Napoca, Romania; negrea.mihai@gmail.com
8. Faculty of Management, The Bucharest University of Economic Studies, 020021 Bucharest, Romania; laurabostangiu@yahoo.com
* Correspondence: popovici.sonia@yahoo.com (S.E.P.); bratu.lavinia@umft.ro (L.M.B.); Tel.: +40-728-001-971
† The authors have equal contribution.

Abstract: The development of general anesthesia techniques and anesthetic substances has opened new horizons for the expansion and improvement of surgical techniques. Nevertheless, more complex surgical procedures have brought a higher complexity and longer duration for general anesthesia, which has led to a series of adverse events such as hemodynamic instability, under- or overdosage of anesthetic drugs, and an increased number of post-anesthetic events. In order to adapt the anesthesia according to the particularities of each patient, the multimodal monitoring of these patients is highly recommended. Classically, general anesthesia monitoring consists of the analysis of vital functions and gas exchange. Multimodal monitoring refers to the concomitant monitoring of the degree of hypnosis and the nociceptive-antinociceptive balance. By titrating anesthetic drugs according to these parameters, clinical benefits can be obtained, such as hemodynamic stabilization, the reduction of awakening times, and the reduction of postoperative complications. Another important aspect is the impact on the status of inflammation and the redox balance. By minimizing inflammatory and oxidative impact, a faster recovery can be achieved that increases patient safety. The purpose of this literature review is to present the most modern multimodal monitoring techniques to discuss the particularities of each technique.

Keywords: hypnosis; multimodal monitoring; entropy; qNOX; qCON; bispectral index; surgical plethysmographic index; general anesthesia; patient safety

1. Introduction

The rapid developments in the field of anesthesia, including new drugs, new anesthetic techniques, and new monitoring devices, have led to an increased trust in the anesthetic act from the general population and increased addressability toward surgical services, also promoting the development of more complex surgical techniques. In order to keep up with the demand multiparametric monitoring techniques in general anesthesia, rapid adaption is needed. This would lead to shorter waiting times, less post-operatory adverse events, and an increase in patient safety [1–9].

The state of consciousness is represented by a series of variables that can be experienced and felt, such as perceptions, sensations, emotions, and memories, making the quantitative analysis of these states impossible. One of the first state-of-consciousness theories launched in 1949 by Hebb, who postulated that the physical transposition of a mental representation is given by the neuro-cellular assembly and by the neuronal interconnections [5]. The N-metil-D-aspartate (NMDA) synapses were discovered based on this first theory, and after numerous studies, researchers found that synapses are predominantly found in the cortex [6–8]. Diverse interactions, ionic exchanges, the production of nitric oxide, and the electrical stimulation generated by the opening and closing of ion channels leads to the formation of inter-neuronal connections and to a complex neuronal activity. The loss of consciousness can have a number of causes, such as anesthesia, cerebral lesions, or sleep. In the case of anesthesia, the responses of the central nervous system are totally suppressed. This state is reversible, and it is an attribute of the development of modern medicine that has enabled the development of modern surgery and invasive therapeutic and diagnostic techniques [10–25].

Multimodal monitoring techniques in general anesthesia refer to the utilization of all parameters that characterize this process. Therefore, we talk about monitoring of the degree of hypnosis, of the nociception-antinociception balance, and of the functionality of the autonomic nervous system [23]. In the classical state of things, general anesthesia monitoring includes the evaluation of vital functions such as heart rate, blood pressure, temperature, and other subjective clinical findings. In this situation, there is always a risk of under- or overdosage of anesthetics, leading to either awareness or an excessive degree of hypnosis, with serious impact on the outcome and prognosis of these patients. Clinical signs such as hypertension, tachycardia, and tearing have long been used for guiding general anesthesia, but it has already been proven that they are subjective and cannot guide general anesthesia in an individualized manner, in accordance with the real needs of each patient [2,24,25].

Electroencephalography (EEG) is the recording of postsynaptic potentials in the pyramidal cells of the cerebral cortex. EEG is classified then based on the frequency. It can be recorded on the scalp and forehead using surface electrodes and reflects the metabolic activity of the brain. The metabolic activity of brain cells needs energy. Problems or changes in energy production (increased demand or decrease production) by brain cells can profoundly affect EEG activity [10–12]. Monitoring of the level of consciousness during general anesthesia based on electroencephalography has become a routine practice in the operating room. Both for the patient and anesthetist, the main concern during general anesthesia is the state of unconsciousness, mainly avoiding the risk of awareness. EEG models are well known to change in pattern with the deepening of anesthesia. Therefore, evaluating the degree of hypnosis requires measurements of the electrical activity of the brain [13–15]. The brain is the target effect site of anesthetics. Therefore, the brain needs to be monitored together with spinal reflexes and cardiovascular changes such as mean arterial pressure and heart rate. Measuring the depth of anesthesia is based on continuous EEG monitoring. Certain algorithms have been developed able to translate changes in the EEG signals into simple numerical indices that correspond to a certain level of anesthesia, from awake state to deep sleep [3,16,17]. Monitoring the state of consciousness is a complex endeavor and, although this clinical area has evolved rapidly, the benefits of EEG monitoring-based anesthesia are still controversial. The problem lies in the fact that our understanding of the human consciousness state is still incomplete, and we still lack information about the exact effects of general anesthesia on the brain. The depth of anesthesia is neither stable nor constant. Instead, it is more of a dynamic action that depends on the balance between the dosage of anesthetic medication and the pain caused by the surgical intervention [18–20].

Using EEG signal in order to monitor the depth of general anesthesia should reduce the incidence of intra-anesthetic awareness, lead to a reduction in anesthetic medication consumption, reduce the incidence of adverse effects related to anesthesia, and lead to shorter recovery times [21,22].

2. Multimodal Monitoring Techniques for the Degree of Hypnosis

In the current clinical practice, achieving an individualized prediction of the response to sedation and hypnosis is not accurate without multiparametric monitoring because of complex factors and variables that interfere with the anesthetic act. Among these, the most common are the concomitant administration of anesthetic agents, as well as the different pharmacokinetic response and the individual pharmacodynamic variability. Therefore, real-time monitoring of the effects induced by general anesthesia can bring an important contribution to the optimization of anesthetic dosage and hemodynamic control by the individualized titration of these medications. In order to limit perioperative adverse effects induced by the anesthetic drugs, it is recommended to titrate the doses based on the individual clinical response [26–28]. Some of the most common techniques for the evaluation and quantification of the degree of hypnosis are represented by the bispectral index (BIS, Medtronic-Covidien, Dublin, Ireland), Entropy (GE Healthcare, Helsinki, Finland), composite auditory evoked potential index (cAAI, AEP Monitor/2, Danmeter A/S, Odense, Denmark), and Narcotrend index (NCT, MonitorTechnik, Germany).

Bispectral analysis is a statistical technique that reveals nonlinear phenomena such as the electroencephalogram (EEG). The conventional analysis of EEG signals using standard procedures can bring important information regarding the frequency, power, and phase of EEG signals. The bispectral analysis of these signals represents a separate technique that analyses sinusoidal segments of the EEG spectrum, showing quantifiable variables in the form of an index (BIS) with clinical applicability. From a practical viewpoint, BIS is represented by a numeric interval between 0 and 100, where 0 represents the complete electrical abolition translated through cortical suppression and 100 is characterized by the conscious (awake) state on the EEG [29].

Another technique used for monitoring and individualizing the degree of hypnosis in patients undergoing general anesthesia is Narcotrend (Monitor Technik, Bad Bramstedt, Germany). Narcotrend is based on analyzing the EEG signal, and it classifies the degree of hypnosis in different levels, such as A (awake) and F (electrical silence), quantified by the Narcotrend Index, which ranges from 100 (awake) to 0 (electrical silence) [30]. In a study that compared the performance of the BIS and Narcotrend Index, Kreuer et al. reported similar effects of the two techniques. This research group obtained a prediction probability, P(K), for Narcotrend of 0.88 ± 0.03, while the P(K) for BIS was 0.85 ± 0.04. Furthermore, the mean drug effect, k(e0), was 0.2 ± 0.05 min^{-1} for Narcotrend and 0.16 ± 0.07 min^{-1} for BIS [31]. A similar study was carried out by Kreuer et al., who also reported similarities between the two techniques. Their study included 50 patients undergoing orthopedic surgery and reported statistically significant correlations between the D and E segments of Narcotrend and the 64–40 range of BIS [32]. Another study on the impact of hypnosis monitoring by Narcotrend Index in the pediatric patient population reported strong correlations between the Narcotrend Index and the minimum alveolar concentration (MAC) in patients over 4 months of age [33].

The Auditory evoked potentials (AEPs) represent another technique used for monitoring the degree of hypnosis in patients under general anesthesia [34]. Mantzaridis et al. studied the AEPs Index in patients undergoing orthopedic surgery. The mean value for the index at the beginning of surgery was 72.5 ± 11.2, followed by a decrease to 39.6 ± 6.9 that correlated with loss of consciousness. After recovery from anesthesia, the mean value for the AEPs Index was 66.9 ± 12.5, leading to the conclusion that this index is suitable for being used in the current medical practice [35].

On the other hand, the concept of Entropy derives from thermodynamics and is successfully used in the current clinical practice, with applications in EEG signal analysis. Regarding the mechanism of analysis, the EEG signal is first analyzed based on the "Fast Fourier" [28–31] concept for the identification of the sinusoidal compounds. After identifying the spectra, the Shannon function is applied in order to identify the specific values for each identified frequency. The sum of these values results in the numerical values called Spectral Entropy. The first algorithm ever to be used in the clinical practice has been defined and applied in the M-Entropy modules S/5 (GE Healthcare, Helsinki, Finland) [10,29–45]. The EEG data are collected through an adhesive sensor made of three electrodes applied on the fronto-temporal region. Applying this concept for general anesthesia led to the idea that when the brain is in the "awake status," the EEG signals are complex and present, with a high degree of irregularity. When the patient is asleep/under general anesthesia, the neuronal activity progressively decreases, and the EEG complexes become more regular. Applying the principle in the case of Entropy in patients under general anesthesia, a significant difference has been observed regarding the wave spectrum generated, with this wave spectrum being directly proportional with the neuronal activity. Because the EEG signals are measured from electrodes placed on the frontal region, a high number of signals are represented by the activity of the muscles from the forehead region and are translated though an electromyography signal (EMG). Therefore, the EEG signals are defined by frequencies up to 32 Hz, while the EMG activity includes signals above 32 Hz. The M-Entropy module (GE Healthcare, Helsinki, Finland) distinguishes these two frequencies and generates two different parameters, both having important clinical significance—State Entropy (SE) and Response Entropy (RE). SE (0.8–32 Hz) reflects the cortical status of the patient, while RE (0.8–47 Hz) includes both the EEG and the EMG activity [12,34–36]. The values of SE are between 0 (suppressed EEG) and 91 ("awake status"), while RE is characterized by values between 0–100. In clinical practice, it is recommended to maintain RE/SE between 40 and 60 in order to achieve an adequate degree of hypnosis. Spectral Entropy is based on the analysis of frontal EEG and EMG variations and is a safe and reliable method for monitoring the depth of anesthesia. The Entropy module transforms the irregular content of the EEG signal in an index that reflects the depth of anesthesia. Normally, the signal is acquired from the skin on the forehead and temporal. Hence, it encompasses both an EEG and an EMG component [37]. The index is then calculated based on the following: High levels of entropy during anesthesia demonstrate awareness, while very low entropy levels are correlated with a profound state of unconsciousness. Using this parameter will lead to a more rapid awakening of the patient at the end of surgery and a lower dosage of anesthetic drugs. At the same time, it will prevent intra-anesthetic awareness episodes [32,38–40].

Changes in neuronal activity can be analyzed indirectly through computed tomography with integrated positron emission (PET-CT). This analysis is based on the changes in certain variables, such as neuronal activity, cerebral blood flow, and cellular metabolism [41]. Thus, specific changes in the glucose metabolism rate and cerebral blood flow can be quantified using [^{18}F]–fluorodeoxiglucose and [^{15}O] H_2O. General anesthetic agents such as sevoflurane and propofol reduce the cerebral blood flow, with this effect being more important in the case of propofol. Maksimow et al. carried out a study regarding the changes in neuronal activity under general anesthesia and mapped the cerebral areas that better correlated with the EEG signals. The analysis of the regional cerebral blood flow was studied at different degrees of hypnosis measured by the Minimum Alveolar Concentration (MAC). In particular, the authors used MAC:1, MAC:1.5, and MAC:2 for sevoflurane, and different half maximal effective concentrations for propofol (EC50) at 30 min intervals. For patients in the sevoflurane group, the authors analyzed the End-Tidal Sevoflurane (Et-Sevo): 0% Et-Sevo (patient awake), 2% Et-Sevo (1 MAC), 3% Et-Sevo (1.5 MAC), and 4% Et-Sevo (2 MAC), while for the propofol group the analyzed group, the authors measured

0 microg/mL (patient awake), 6 microg/mL (1 EC50), 9 microg/mL (1.5 EC50), and 12 microg/mL (2 EC50). In both groups, the Entropy was inversely proportional with the sevoflurane and propofol concentrations, with reductions from 73.5 ± 6.5 to 12.2 ± 9.4 and from 70.4 ± 7.1 to 0.6 ± 1, respectively, in the frontal region. In the temporo-occipital region, the Entropy analysis was similar, following the same dose-dependent trend. Regarding the correlation between EEG/SE analysis and computed tomography, the researchers found statistically significant correlations for both drugs at similar concentrations (1.5 MAC, $r = 0.81$ și 1.5 EC50, $r = 0.83$). Following this study, Maksimow et al. validated the fact that spectral Entropy can be used for both sevoflurane and propofol, showing the same regional neuronal activity confirmed through noninvasive PET-CT analysis. The usage of monitoring techniques for the degree of hypnosis in the case of pediatric patients is limited and is not validated. Numerous studies have analyzed the statistical correlations between BIS and Entropy for different age groups but have not identified strong statistical correlations between BIS/Entropy values and anesthetic drugs concentrations in infants vs. pediatric patients (aged over 1 year old) [42]. Davidson et al. carried out a study regarding the performance of BIS and Entropy for different age groups in pediatric patients. They analyzed four age groups: 0–1 years old ($n = 8$), 1–2 years old ($n = 10$), 2–4 years old ($n = 18$), and 4–12 years old ($n = 14$). Regarding the comparison between Entropy and BIS, above the initial status (awake), they identified statistically significant differences in the 0–1 years old group, as follows: RE/BIS: 45 vs. 84, $p = 0.003$, SE/BIS: 36 vs. 78 ($p = 0.02$). Following this study, no statistically significant differences have been proven for BIS or for Entropy, especially in the 0–1 age group. Interestingly, there were no performance differences between BIS and Entropy but applying these techniques in the case of infants should be done with caution. In Table 1, a series of implications for different monitoring techniques for the degree of hypnosis on the clinical prognostic of patients undergoing general anesthesia are summarized [43].

Table 1. The impact of monitoring the degree of hypnosis on anesthetic drugs consumption and on time recovery.

Author	Parameter/Monitoring Technique	Type of General Anesthesia	Observations	Reference
Kim et al.	State Entropy (SE)	78 children (age: 3–12) Sevoflurane	↓ sevoflurane consumption ↓ postoperative recovery time	[44]
Wu et al.	State Entropy (SE)	64 patients Sevoflurane	↓ sevoflurane consumption ↓ consumption of antihypertensive drugs ↑ hemodynamic stability	[45]
Vakkuri et al.	State Entropy (SE)	368 patients propofol-alfentanil-N_2O	↓ propofol consumption ↓ postoperative recovery time	[46]
Talawar et al.	Entropy (SE/RE)	50 patients isofluran-N_2O	↓ postoperative recovery time	[47]
Elgebaly et al.	Entropy (SE/RE)	propofol	↓ propofol consumption ↑ hemodynamic stability	[48]
Gan et al.	Bispectral index (BIS)	302 patients propofol-alfentanil-N_2O	↓ propofol consumption ↓ postoperative recovery time	
Liu et al.	Bispectral index (BIS)	1383 patients Day surgery	↓ consumption of anesthetic drugs ↓ incidence of adverse effects (nausea, vomiting) ↓ postoperative recovery time	
Bhardwaj et al.	Bispectral index (BIS)	50 pediatric pts propofol	No effects have been observed regarding the consumption of anesthetic drugs No effects on the postoperative recovery time	[49]

Table 1. *Cont.*

Author	Parameter/Monitoring Technique	Type of General Anesthesia	Observations	Reference
Aime et al.	Bispectral index (BIS) and Entropy (RE/SE)	115 patients Sevoflurane;	BIS & Entropy: ↓ sevoflurane consumption	[50]
Liao et al.	Bispectral index (BIS) and A-line autoregressive index (AAI)	116 patients Sevoflurane;	BIS & AAI: ↓ sevoflurane consumption ↓ postoperative recovery time;	[51]
Weber et al.	Composite auditory evoked potential index (cAAI)	20 pediatric patients TIVA propofol and remifentanil;	↓ propofol consumption ↑ hemodynamic stability	[52]
Lai et al.	Narcotrend	40 patients propofol and fentanyl;	↓ propofol consumption ↓ postoperative recovery time No effects on PONV	[53]
Rundshagen et al.	Narcotrend	48 patients propofol and remifentanil	No effects on propofol/remifentanil consumption No effects on postoperative recovery time	[54]

RE: Response Entropy; SE: State Entropy; BIS: Bispectral Index; TIVA: Total Intravenous Anesthesia; PONV: Postoperative nausea and vomiting; AAI: A-line Autoregresive index; cAAI; composite auditory evoked potential index.

One other widely discussed risk is the incidence of intraoperative awareness that can lead to long-term posttraumatic stress disorder. Sebel et al. carried out a study on the incidence of intra-anesthetic awareness analyzing 19,575 patients. They identified 25 patients that presented with awareness, resulting in an incidence of 0.13%. This research group did not find any statistically significant differences regarding the incidence based on sex or age, but increased incidence was associated with higher The American Society of Anesthesiologists (ASA) physical status classification system scores (odds ratio, 2.41; 95% CI, 1.04–5.60 ASA III–V vs. ASA I–II) [55]. Sebel et al. estimated a rough number of 26,000 cases of intra-anesthetic awareness annually in the United States, and this number is reported to be approximately 20 million among general anesthesia procedures [55]. In a similar study, Bruhn et al. reported an incidence of 0.11% out of 10,811 patients [34]. Ekman et al. reported a 0.18% incidence of awareness in a retrospective study that included 7826 patients [56]. For all listed studies, the incidence of awareness was lower in the groups of patients where techniques for monitoring the degree of hypnosis were used [34,55,56].

3. Monitoring Techniques for the Nociception-Antinociception Balance

Another important aspect in the clinical practice is represented by the continuous monitoring of the nociception-antinociception balance. The aim of these parameters is to aid the clinician in deciding the adequate analgesia dosage for each patient. Whereas monitoring the degree of hypnosis is achieved through the direct evaluation of the EEG signals, the nociception-antinociception balance can be monitored indirectly [9,12] by evaluating certain variables such as the vasomotor reflex, pupillary size, the H reflex, and the hemodynamic response [57,58] (Figure 1).

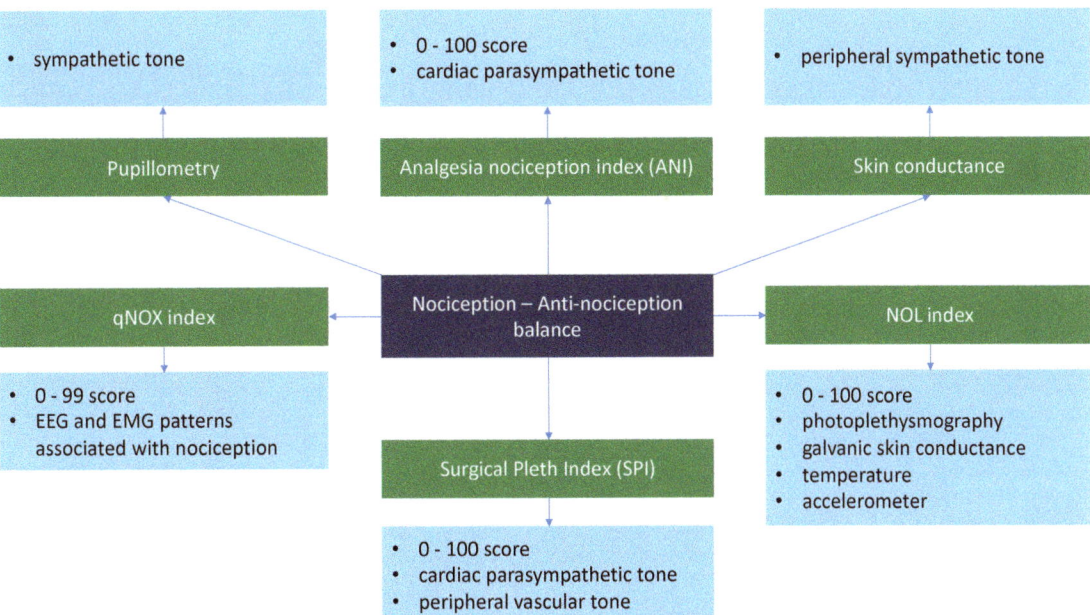

Figure 1. Technologies/parameters used for monitoring the nociception-antinociception balance [59–66]. ANI—analgesia nociception index; qNOX index—index of nociception; SPI—Surgical Plethysmographic Index; NOL index—Nociception Level Index; EEG—Electroencephalography; EMG—Electromyography signal.

One of the most widely studied technologies is the analysis of hemodynamic changes, including the evaluation of the normalized heartbeat intervals (HBIs) and of the amplitude of the plethysmographic waves, both correlating with sympathetic and parasympathetic tones. A higher sympathetic tone correlates with the intensity of the surgical stimuli and results in a suppressed plethysmographic amplitude (PPGA). For the correct calculation of the Surgical Plethysmographic Index (SPI), after normalizing these parameters by transforming the histogram, the SPI formula is used where SPI = 100 − (0.67 × PPGA$_{norm}$ + 0.33 × HBI$_{norm}$). The SPI value can be influenced by certain factors, such as cardiac pacemakers, cardiac arrhythmias, antiarrhythmic medication, beta−1 adrenergic antagonists, and alpha2-adrenergic agonists. Bonhomme et al. evaluated the Surgical Pleth Index (SPI, GE Healthcare, Helsinki, Finland) trend and made correlations with variability in mean arterial pressure and heartrate. Following this study, they showed that there is a strong correlation between all these variables. Therefore SPI values depend on the doses of opioid medication administered during the anesthesia [58]. Bergmann et al. carried out a randomized study that included 170 patients receiving general anesthesia with propofol and remifentanil. The patients were divided in two study groups. One study group received opioids based on SPI values, while the other group received the doses of opioids based on standard monitoring parameters, both clinical and hemodynamic monitoring. Statistically significant differences were shown in both propofol ($p < 0.05$, 6.0 ± 2.1 vs. 7.5 ± 2.2 mg/kg/h) and remifentanil ($p < 0.05$, 0.06 ± 0.04 vs. 0.08 ± 0.05 µg/kg/min) consumption. The impact on post-anesthesia recovery time was evaluated by the time needed to open the eyes and time to extubation. The results presented statistical significance for both the evaluated features, extubation time ($p < 0.05$, 1.2 ± 4.4 min vs. 4.4 ± 4.5 min), and eye-opening time ($p < 0.05$, −0.08 ± 4.4 min vs. 3.5 ± 4.3 min). The conclusion was that dose reduction and shorter recovery times can be achieved by adapting general anesthesia based on the SPI [10]. Huiku et al. confirmed in a similar study that SPI monitoring has a beneficial impact on anesthetic drugs used doses, increasing patient safety and the quality of the medical services [67].

Another parameter used for the evaluation of the nociception-antinociception balance is the Analgesia Nociception Index (ANI) [68]. The technology is based on the assessment in heart rate variability. In the clinical setting, ANI values lie between 0 and 100. In this case, 0 represents a very low degree of parasympathetic modulation and 100 represent a very high degree of parasympathetic activity. From a clinical point of view, ANI = 0 represents high stress levels, while ANI = 100 represents low stress levels.

Dostalova et al. carried out a study in which they compared the impact the two monitoring techniques have on general anesthesia. They had three study groups: The group where doses of opioids were titrated based on ANI values, the SPI group, and the control group. They showed statistically significant differences regarding the decrease in opioid consumption and shorter recovery times after anesthesia [68]. Table 2 summarizes a series of studies regarding the impact of monitoring techniques on the nociception-antinociception balance and on the clinical outcome of patients.

Table 2. The impact of nociception-antinociception monitoring techniques on anesthetic drugs consumption and on recovery time.

Author	Technique/ Parameter	Type of Anesthesia Type of Intervention	Obervations	Reference
Funcke et al.	SPI & Pupillary Pain Index (PPI) & Nociception Level (NOL)	48 patients radical retropubic prostatectomy	SPI: ↓ hormonal response to stress PPI: ↓ sufentanil consumption, ↑ hormonal response to stress No effect on postoperative recovery time	[69]
Bergmann et al.	Surgical Pleth Index (SPI)	170 patients orthopedic surgery	↓ propofol consumption ↓ remifentanil consumption ↓ postoperative recovery time	[10]
Jain et al.	Surgical Pleth Index (SPI)	140 patients Laparoscopic cholecystectomy;	↓ PONV ↓ postoperative pain ↑ fentanyl consumption No impact on hemodynamic stability	[70]
Won et al.	Surgical Pleth Index (SPI)	45 patient; Elective thyroidectomy	↓ oxycodone consumption ↓ postoperative recovery time ↓ extubation time	[71]
Chen et al.	Surgical Stress Index (SSI)–former Surgical Pleth Index (SPI)	80 patients Elective surgical interventions	↓ remifentanil consumption ↓ postoperative adverse effects ↑ hemodynamic stability	[72]
Theerth et al.	Analgesia Nociception Index (ANI)	60 patients Oncological surgery	↓ fentanyl consumption No impact on postoperative pain	[73]
Soral et al.	Analgesia Nociception Index (ANI)	102 patients Procedural sedation	↓ opioid consumption No impact of propofol and ketamine consumption	[74]
Gall et al.	Analgesia Nociception Index (ANI)	60 patients Bariatric surgery	↓ sufentanyl consumption No impact on PONV and postoperative pain	[75]

Numerous studies have shown that opioid overdose during anesthesia is responsible for a series of adverse effects, such as increased recovery times and opioid induced hyperalgesia, and that opioid overdose also leads to hypotension, having a major impact on perioperative hemodynamic stability [66–71]. Won et al. reported that using SPI monitoring during general anesthesia reduced opioid consumption, improved hemodynamic stability, and reduced postoperative recovery times [71]. A similar study was carried out by Jain et al., which showed a statistically significant decrease in the number of hemodynamic adverse events when SPI was used for the titration of opioid medication ($p < 0.05$) [70].

Another system used for monitoring the nociception-antinociception balance is the index of nociception (qNOX) (qCON 2000 Monitor, Quantium Medical, Fresenius Kabi, Mataro, Spain). This parameter is based on the evaluation of EEG and EMG patterns, with values between 0 and 99. Jensen et al. carried out a study on 60 patients undergoing general anesthesia with propofol and remifentanil and showed a series of statistically significant correlations, concluding that qNOX can detect fine changes in the nociception-antinociception balance [76]. The Nociception Level Index (NOL Index, Medasense, Ramat Gau, Israel) is another widely used technology for titrating analgesic drugs during general anesthesia. It analyses the photoplethysmographic wave, temperature, skin galvanic conductance response, and accelerometry [63].

4. The Impact of Multimodal Monitoring on the Hemodynamic Status

During general anesthesia, maintaining adequate tissue perfusion represents one of the most important goals in the perioperative management of the patient. Hypotension frequently occurs, especially after the induction of anesthesia, that is, between the moment of induction and the start of surgery. Reich et al. reported a decrease in mean arterial pressure (MAP) of over 40% (MAP < 70mmHg or MAP < 60 mmHg) in the first 10 min after induction ($p < 0.001$) [77]. Moreover, this study ($n = 2406$ patients) reported an increase in the time spent in the recovery room (13.3%, $p < 0.05$) and in postoperative mortality rates (8.6%, $p < 0.02$) in patients that presented perioperative hypotension. Another interesting phenomenon presented by the group was that post-induction hypotension was more frequent in the 5–10 min interval in comparison to the 0–5 min interval after induction of general anesthesia [77]. A similar study carried out by Hug et al. reported that over 15% of patients presented a decrease in systolic blood pressure (SBP) under 90 mmHg after induction with propofol in the first 10 min after administration [78]. Studies have shown that induction with sevoflurane maintains hemodynamic stability and decreases the risk of hypotension in comparison to induction with propofol, as this technique is not as well tolerated by the patients. Thwaites et al. studied the satisfaction of patients regarding the induction technique used: Sevoflurane (inhalational induction, 8%) vs. propofol (i.v. induction). Over 14% of the patients considered inhalational induction unpleasant in comparison to 10% in the case of propofol. Furthermore, over 24% of the patients would not choose sevoflurane induction the second time [79].

Cerebral ischemia is one of the main causes for cognitive impairment, with a very high global degree of mortality, while motor and cognitive dysfunctions seriously affect the quality of life of these patients. Cerebral reperfusion after an ischemic episode can induce organ damage such as neurovascular injury, neuronal death, cerebral edema, and neuro-hemorrhagic changes. The most common cellular mechanisms involved are represented by apoptosis, inflammation, and excessive production of free radicals [80].

The impact of hypotension during general anesthesia on the postoperative outcome and on the development of postoperative adverse events has been widely studied. Intraoperative hypotension (IHO) is a common effect of general anesthesia and has been associated with an increased incidence of 1-year mortality after surgery [81,82].

The most important predictors for perioperative morbidity and mortality are the associated comorbidities, the determinants of the surgical procedure, and the specific aspects of perioperative management and of general anesthesia. Apart from monitoring the hemodynamic parameters, quantification of the degree of hypnosis "depth of anesthesia" represents one of the most important parameters in modern general anesthesia. At the time, monitoring the degree of hypnosis is possible using techniques based on the analysis of electroencephalography signals (EEG) [83].

Monk et al. studied the 1-year prognosis of patients that underwent noncardiac surgery under general anesthesia. The research group carried out complex statistical analysis in order to determine if death at 1 year after can be associated with significant clinical features of the patient or with the management of general anesthesia. In order to control the degree of hypnosis, they used the Bispectral Index ® (BIS®), with the same type of electrodes for all patients included in the study (A1050BIS Monitor, BIS sensors, Aspect Medical Systems, Newton, MA).

Global mortality at 1 year was 5.5% ($n = 1604$) and 10.3% for patients aged over 65 ($n = 243$). Regarding the variables that correlate with mortality, Monk et al. reported three statistically significant segments: 1. Patient comorbidities (relative risk 6.116, $p < 0.05$); 2. General anesthesia overdosage/deep anesthesia, BIS < 45 (relative risk 1.244/h, $p < 0.05$); 3. Systolic hypotension during surgery (relative risk 1.036/min, $p < 0.05$) [83]. They concluded that prolonged intraoperative hypotension can be associated with an increased incidence in mortality at 1 year [83]. Although numerous studies have focused on perioperative hypotension, at the time there, is no clear definition for IHO [84]. Most of the studies have addressed the statistical associations and correlations between different numerical intervals and correlations with the clinical changes. Sun et al. carried out a study on the impact of IHO on acute kidney injury (AKI). Furthermore, the research group investigated the implications IHO time have on the incidence of AKI. They correlated the AKI incidence with different IHO intervals as follows: MAP < 55 mmHg, MAP < 60 mmHg, and MAP < 65 mmHg [85]. This was a retrospective study that included 5127 patients between 2009 and 2012. The results showed an AKI incidence of 6.3% (324 patients) for MAP < 60 mmHg and an IHO time between 11–20 min, and MAP < 55 for an IHO time >10 min. Sun et al. reported a strong statistical correlation between sustained episodes of IHO with a MAP < 50 mmHg and MAP < 60 mmHg and AKI incidence. For the evaluation of AKI, they considered a 50% increase in creatinine levels or 0.3 mg/dL in the first 2 days after surgery. A similar study was developed by Walsh et al. regarding the implications of IHO on the incidence of AKI and myocardial injury. They evaluated 33,330 patients that had undergone noncardiac surgery, making statistical correlations between the incidence of AKI and myocardial injury in patients that presented with IHO with a MAP < 55 mmHg and MAP < 75 mmHg. Following statistical analysis, they identified 2478 patients that had developed AKI (7.4%) and 770 (2.3%) with myocardial injuries. For both groups, MAP was under 55 mmHg. Interestingly, the risk for developing renal and myocardial lesions was increased, even for short IHO times [86]. In a similar context, a metanalysis carried out by Wesselink et al. reported ischemic organ damage when MAP < 80 mmHg for longer than 10 min. This research group showed an increase in risk with any decrease in blood pressure [84].

5. The Impact of General Anesthesia Multimodal Monitoring on Inflammation/Redox

Another important aspect that also has an impact on the clinical outcome of surgical patients is represented by the inflammatory status and the oxidoreduction response (REDOX) [87–91]. The excessive production of free nitrogen and oxygen radicals has a direct involvement in the augmentation of the pro-inflammatory status. Under physiological conditions, the balance between the production of free radicals and that of endogenous antioxidant substances maintains the oxidoreduction equilibrium and the body does not suffer. Under surgical stress, in the case of ischemia-reperfusion syndrome or hypotension, an excessive number of free radicals will be produced, as well as proinflammatory mediators. All these factors will also decrease the production capacity for antioxidant molecules [92].

Particularly in the case of patients under GA (general anesthesia) or in mechanically ventilated patients, oxygen plays an essential role in therapeutic management. In the case of general anesthesia, increased oxygen inspiratory fractions (FiO$_2$) are administered before endotracheal intubation and after extubation in order to maintain an adequate oxygen plasma concentration. Under physiological conditions, P$_a$O$_2$ = 80–100 mmHg. When P$_a$O$_2$ exceeds 100 mmHg, the patient is characterized by hyperoxia, the most important systemic effect being the increased and accelerated production of reactive oxygen species (ROS) and the development of oxidative stress (OS) [93–99]. The most important mechanisms through which OS is augmented in the case of general anesthesia are represented by the increase in molecular oxygen offerings at the mitochondria, the interaction with reactive nitrogen species (RNS), and lipid peroxidation with destruction of cellular membranes [25,100–103] (Figure 2).

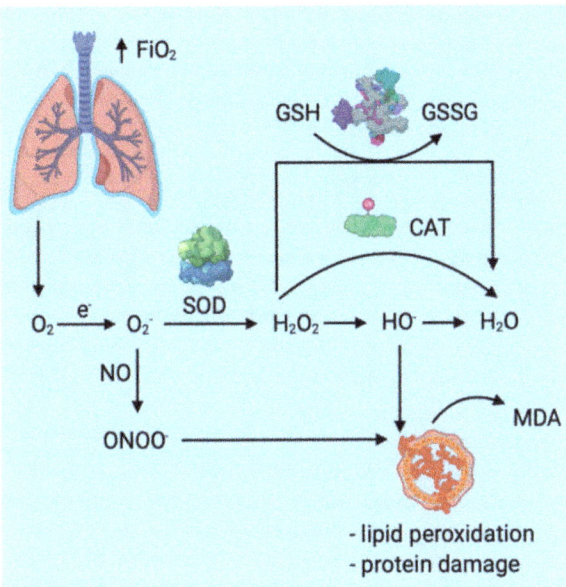

Figure 2. Schematic representation of the oxidative response in patients under general anesthesia.

Nunes et al. studied the implications of general anesthesia (GA) on the redox profile of surgical patients that underwent intravenous GA, as well as the implications of multimodal monitoring based on Entropy on the oxidoreduction activity. The study included 20 patients divided into 2 study groups. In the first group, the Entropy values were maintained in the 45–59 interval, and in the second, Entropy was maintained in the 30–44 interval in order to evaluate the impact of anesthetic overdosage on the redox balance. The patients were evaluated at different moments in time: M1—right after the administration of anesthetic drugs, M2—after endotracheal intubation, M3—5 min after endotracheal intubation, M4—immediately after surgical pneumoperitoneum, M5—1 min after pneumoperitoneum, and M6—1 h after the end of surgery. The researchers determined the plasma concentrations for Glutathione and TBARS (tiobarbituric acid reactive species). Following the analysis, they identified significant increases in the Glutathione and TBARS concentrations at M5 in both groups. There were statistically significant differences between the two study groups, with higher values of both Glutathione and TBARS in the group where Entropy was maintained between 30 and 44 ($p < 0.05$). In regard to the anesthetic management, recovery times were significantly shorter for the group where Entropy levels were kept between 45 and 59 (7.70 ± 1.24 min vs. 10.20 ± 0.90 min, $p < 0.05$). The increase in redox imbalance markers for the patients that received a deeper hypnosis (Entropy 20–44) reveals an increase in anaerobic metabolism, possibly because of an accentuated suppression of the autonomic nervous system [92].

Ferrari et al. carried out a study regarding the genotoxicity of sevoflurane on the DNA structure in isolated lymphocytes in 20 patients undergoing orthopedic surgery under GA. They showed important changes in DNA structure and in redox activity that correlated statistically with the sevoflurane concentration [104]. Compared to the exposure to propofol, the group that was exposed to sevoflurane presented a marked increase in the expression of tumor necrosis factor alpha (TNF-alpha) and a decrease for interleukin 10 (IL-10) [104,105].

6. The Impact of Multiparametric Monitoring on Drug Consumption and Recovery

Gan et al. led an important study regarding the implications of monitoring the degree of hypnosis. They included 302 patients divided in 2 groups. In the study group, GA was guided based on BIS monitoring, while in the control group, anesthesia was guided with basic monitoring. BIS values were measured in both groups [106]. In the study group, the dosage of anesthetic agents was optimized in order to achieve a mean BIS value between 40 and 60 based on current guidelines and recommendations. Interestingly enough, the BIS values in the control group were under 40, indicating a tendency to overdose the anesthetic agents. The total propofol consumption was lower in the study group compared to the control. Another important variable was the time to extubation, which was 7.27 min shorter (95% CI 6.23–8.28 min) in the study group compared to 11.22 min in the control group (95% CI, 8.51–13.60 min). Song et al. designed a similar study that also showed a decrease in extubation times in patients that received general anesthesia modulated based on BIS, with a reduction from 6.5 ± 4.3 min to 3.6 ± 1.5 min (>40%) for Desflurane, and from 7.7 ± 3.5 min to 5.5 ± 2.2 min for sevoflurane [107].

Vakkuri et al. carried out a multicenter study on the impact the monitoring of degree of hypnosis through Entropy (GE Healthcare, Helsinki, Finland) has on anesthetic drug consumption and on postoperative recovery time. In the final analysis of the study, they included 308 patients, divided homogeneously in 2 groups: The control group and the study group, where GA was modulated based on Entropy. For propofol consumption, there were statistically significant differences between the two study groups, with the median for the control group being 0.11 (0.03, 0.21) mg/kg/min vs. 0.10 (0.04, 0.23) mg/kg/min for the group where Entropy was used.

The analysis of the implications multimodal monitoring has on the postoperative recovery showed a decrease in the time to spontaneous breathing in the study group (4.74 (0.00, 18.0) minutes) compared to the median in the control group (7.07 (1.00–28.5) minutes). Using Entropy also decreased the time to extubation from 9.16 (1.67, 32.3) minutes to 5.80 (3.00, 27.3) minutes, with $p <0.05$. The patients in the target group opened their eyes to verbal command faster than the control group (6.08 (0.15, 37.5) minutes vs. 10.8 (2.23, 43.2) minutes ($p < 0.05$)), and they were transferred to the Post-Anesthesia Care Unit (PACU) faster, at 10.3 (1.17, 48.7, $p < 0.05$) minutes vs. 13.0 (5.0, 49.8) minutes. Mean State Entropy (SE) during general anesthesia was 50 (34–78), while the mean Response Entropy (RE) was 52 (35–84). [46]. A similar study was developed by El Hor et al., reporting an increase in sevoflurane consumption in the case of patients that could not benefit from advanced monitoring of the degree of hypnosis vs. patients for which Entropy monitoring was applied (5.2 ± 1.4 mL/h vs. 3.8 ± 1.5 mL/h, $p < 0.05$) [108]. Regarding hemodynamic stability, the researchers found statistically significant differences between the groups: 10 hypertension episodes were reported in the control group vs. 7 hypertension episodes in the target group. For hypotension, the ratio was 3 in the control group vs. 0 in the target group ($p < 0.05$). Tachycardia episodes were reported as 5 (control group) vs. 8 (target group), while bradycardia episodes were reported as 1 (control group) vs. 0 (study group).

Wu et al. analyzed the impact of multiparametric monitoring based on Entropy (GE Datex-Ohmeda S/5) on the recovery time and anesthetic drugs consumption in patients undergoing orthopedic surgery. This research group included 68 patients in their analysis, divided into 2 groups: The target group with Entropy monitoring and the control group with classical anesthesia monitoring. Sevoflurane consumption was significantly lower in the target group 27.79 ± 7.4 mL/patient vs. 31.42 ± 6.9 mL/patient, $p < 0.05$. Statistically significant differences were also reported for hemodynamic stability, as the target group presented fewer hypertensive episodes compared to the control, 0.94 ± 1.15 vs. 1.48 ± 1.41, $p < 0.05$. Following this study, the research group concluded that using Entropy-based multimodal monitoring significantly reduces both sevoflurane consumption and the consumption of antihypertensive agents [45].

The impact of multiparametric monitoring on the anesthetic drugs consumption was proven in another study by Tewari et al. in patients undergoing gynecological and obstetrical surgery. They analyzed 120 patients that were divided into two study groups based on monitoring technique, with an Entropy group and a classical monitoring of general anesthesia group. They showed that Entropy monitoring led to a reduction of propofol doses (6.7% reduction, p = 0.01), but also that the Fentanyl doses were 10.9% larger in this group (p = 0.07). They did not find any statistically significant differences for recovery time and discharge time from PACU [109–111]. In their study on the impact of Entropy on sevoflurane consumption in major hepatic surgery, Refaat et al. showed a marked decrease in the doses [110].

7. Conclusions

General anesthesia techniques are much more advanced nowadays compared to latter decades, in accordance with the surgical needs and with the needs of the general population. Medical services tend to become more and more complex, managing to solve a wide range of pathologies in all surgical fields. In order to increase both patient safety and medical act quality, as well as to decrease waiting times and to be able to answer the needs of an increasing number of patients, endowment with modern multiparametric monitoring techniques for general anesthesia is necessary. In conclusion, we can state that using monitoring techniques for the degree of hypnosis, the nociception-antinociception balance, and the hemodynamic status markedly increases patient safety. Furthermore, by reducing postoperative recovery times and reducing anesthetic drugs doses, one can highlight the positive impact, both short- and long-term, that multiparametric monitoring has from an economic viewpoint.

Author Contributions: Conceptualization, A.F.R. and D.S.; methodology, D.N.G., M.N., C.M.D. and L.B.P. software, O.H.B.; validation, D.S. and M.P.; formal analysis, A.M. and S.R.; investigation, A.F.R.; resources, C.R.B., A.M.; data curation, L.M.B. and S.E.P.; writing—original draft preparation, A.F.R., S.E.P. and D.T.; writing—review and editing, A.R., L.M.B. and C.M.D.; visualization, D.S.; supervision, D.S.; project administration, O.H.B. and M.P.; funding acquisition, D.S. and A.F.R. All authors have read and agreed to the published version of the manuscript.

Funding: This research received no external funding.

Institutional Review Board Statement: Not applicable.

Informed Consent Statement: Not applicable.

Data Availability Statement: Not applicable.

Conflicts of Interest: The authors declare no conflict of interest.

References

1. Rosenberger, P.; Drexler, B. Development of Anaesthesia-Related Mortality and Impact on Perioperative Outcome. *Anasthesiol. Intensivmed. Notfallmed. Schmerzther.* **2017**, *52*, 486–497. [CrossRef] [PubMed]
2. Guerrero, J.L.; Matute, F.; Alsina, E.; Del Blanco, B.; Gilsanz, F. Response entropy changes after noxius stimulus. *J. Clin. Monit. Comput.* **2012**, *26*, 171–175. [CrossRef] [PubMed]
3. Lehmann, A.; Schmidt, M.; Zeitler, C.; Kiessling, A.-H.; Isgro, F.; Boldt, J. Bispectral index and electroencephalographic entropy in patients undergoing aortocoronary bypass grafting. *Eur. J. Anaesthesiol.* **2007**, *24*, 751–760. [CrossRef] [PubMed]
4. Medical Advisory Secretariat. Bispectral index monitor: An evidence-based analysis. *Ont. Health Technol. Assess. Ser.* **2004**, *4*, 1–70.
5. Hebb, M.O.; McArthur, D.L.; Alger, J.; Etchepare, M.; Glenn, T.C.; Bergsneider, M.; Martin, N.; Vespa, P.M. Impaired percent alpha variability on continuous electroencephalography is associated with thalamic injury and predicts poor long-term outcome after human traumatic brain injury. *J. Neurotrauma* **2007**, *24*, 579–590. [CrossRef] [PubMed]
6. Petras, M.; Tatarkova, Z.; Kovalska, M.; Mokra, D.; Dobrota, D.; Lehotsky, J.; Drgova, A. Hyperhomocysteinemia as a risk factor for the neuronal system disorders. *J. Physiol. Pharmacol.* **2014**, *65*, 15–23. [CrossRef]
7. Sleigh, J.; Harvey, M.; Voss, L.; Denny, B. Ketamine—More mechanisms of action than just NMDA blockade. *Trends Anaesth. Crit. Care* **2014**, *4*, 76–81. [CrossRef]
8. Abushik, P.A.; Niittykoski, M.; Giniatullina, R.; Shakirzyanova, A.; Bart, G.; Fayuk, D.; Sibarov, D.A.; Antonov, S.M.; Giniatullin, R. The role of NMDA and mGluR5 receptors in calcium mobilization and neurotoxicity of homocysteine in trigeminal and cortical neurons and glial cells. *J. Neurochem.* **2014**, *129*, 264–274. [CrossRef]

9. Dinu, A.R.; Rogobete, A.F.; Popovici, S.E.; Bedreag, O.H.; Papurica, M.; Dumbuleu, C.M.; Velovan, R.R.; Toma, D.; Georgescu, C.M.; Trache, L.I.; et al. Impact of general anesthesia guided by state entropy (SE) and response entropy (RE) on perioperative stability in elective laparoscopic cholecystectomy patients—A prospective observational randomized monocentric study. *Entropy* **2020**, *22*, 356. [CrossRef]
10. Bergmann, I.; Göhner, A.; Crozier, T.A.; Hesjedal, B.; Wiese, C.H.; Popov, A.F.; Bauer, M.; Hinz, J.M. Surgical pleth index-guided remifentanil administration reduces remifentanil and propofol consumption and shortens recovery times in outpatient anaesthesia. *Br. J. Anaesth.* **2013**, *110*, 622–628. [CrossRef]
11. Aho, A.J.; Kamata, K.; Jäntti, V.; Kulkas, A.; Hagihira, S.; Huhtala, H.; Yli-Hankala, A. Comparison of Bispectral Index and Entropy values with electroencephalogram during surgical anaesthesia with sevoflurane. *Br. J. Anaesth.* **2015**, *115*, 258–266. [CrossRef] [PubMed]
12. Freye, E.; Levy, J.V. *Cerebral Monitoring in the Operating Room and the Intensive Care Unit: An Introductory for the Clinician and a Guide for the Novice Wanting to Open a Window to the Brain*; Springer: Dordrecht, The Netherlands, 2005; Volume 19, ISBN 1087700507.
13. Klockars, J.G.M.; Hiller, A.; Münte, S.; Van Gils, M.J.; Taivainen, T. Spectral entropy as a measure of hypnosis and hypnotic drug effect of total intravenous anesthesia in children during slow induction and maintenance. *Anesthesiology* **2012**, *116*, 340–351. [CrossRef] [PubMed]
14. Bibian, S.; Dumont, G.A.; Zikov, T. Dynamic behavior of BIS, M-entropy and neuroSENSE brain function monitors. *J. Clin. Monit. Comput.* **2011**, *25*, 81–87. [CrossRef] [PubMed]
15. Shortal, B.P.; Hickman, L.B.; Mak-McCully, R.A.; Wang, W.; Brennan, C.; Ung, H.; Litt, B.; Tarnal, V.; Janke, E.; Picton, P.; et al. Duration of EEG suppression does not predict recovery time or degree of cognitive impairment after general anaesthesia in human volunteers. *Br. J. Anaesth.* **2019**, *123*, 206–218. [CrossRef]
16. Schultz, A.; Siedenberg, M.; Grouven, U.; Kneif, T.; Schultz, B. Comparison of narcotrend index, bispectral index, spectral and entropy parameters during induction of propofol-remifentanil anaesthesia. *J. Clin. Monit. Comput.* **2008**, *22*, 103–111. [CrossRef]
17. Singh, S.; Bansal, S.; Kumar, G.; Gupta, I.; Thakur, J.R. Entropy as an indicator to measure depth of anaesthesia for Laryngeal Mask Airway (LMA) insertion during sevoflurane and propofol anaesthesia. *J. Clin. Diagn. Res.* **2017**, *11*, UC01–UC03. [CrossRef]
18. Iannuzzi, M.; Iannuzzi, E.; Rossi, F.; Berrino, L.; Chiefari, M. Relationship between Bispectral Index, electroencephalographic state entropy and effect-site EC 50 for propofol at different clinical endpoints. *Br. J. Anaesth.* **2005**, *94*, 492–495. [CrossRef]
19. Wildemeersch, D.; Peeters, N.; Saldien, V.; Vercauteren, M.; Hans, G. Pain assessment by pupil dilation reflex in response to noxious stimulation in anaesthetized adults. *Acta Anaesthesiol. Scand.* **2018**, *62*, 1050–1056. [CrossRef]
20. Kumar, A.; Anand, S. A depth of anaesthesia index from linear regression of EEG parameters. *J. Clin. Monit. Comput.* **2006**, *20*, 67–73. [CrossRef]
21. Jagadeesan, N.; Wolfson, M.; Chen, Y.; Willingham, M.; Avidan, M.S. Brain monitoring during general anesthesia. *Trends Anaesth. Crit. Care* **2013**, *3*, 13–18. [CrossRef]
22. Johansen, J.W.; Sebel, P.S. Development and clinical application electroencephalographic bispectrum monitoring. *Anesthesiology* **2000**, *93*, 1336–1344. [CrossRef] [PubMed]
23. Rogobete, A.F.; Bedreag, O.H.; Sandesc, D. Entropy-Guided Depth of Anesthesia in Critically Ill Polytrauma Patients. *J. Interdiscip. Med.* **2017**, *2*, 7–8. [CrossRef]
24. Klockars, J.G.M.; Hiller, A.; Ranta, S.; Talja, P.; Van Gils, M.J.; Taivainen, T. Spectral entropy as a measure of hypnosis in children. *Anesthesiology* **2006**, *104*, 708–717. [CrossRef] [PubMed]
25. Cotae, A.; Grințescu, I.M. Entropy—The Need of an Ally for Depth of Anesthesia Monitoring in Emergency Surgery. *CEACR* **2019**, 13–15. [CrossRef]
26. Lonjaret, L.; Lairez, O.; Minville, V.; Geeraerts, T. Optimal perioperative management of arterial blood pressure. *Integr. Blood Press. Control* **2014**, *7*, 49–59. [CrossRef] [PubMed]
27. Südfeld, S.; Brechnitz, S.; Wagner, J.Y.; Reese, P.C.; Pinnschmidt, H.O.; Reuter, D.A.; Saugel, B. Post-induction hypotension and early intraoperative hypotension associated with general anaesthesia. *Br. J. Anaesth.* **2017**, *119*, 57–64. [CrossRef] [PubMed]
28. Hoppe, P.; Kouz, K.; Saugel, B. Perioperative hypotension: Clinical impact, diagnosis, and therapeutic approaches. *J. Emerg. Crit. Care Med.* **2020**, *4*, 8. [CrossRef]
29. Barnard, J.P.; Bennett, C.; Voss, L.J.; Sleigh, J.W.; Hospital, W.; Zealand, N. Neurosciences and neuroanaesthesia can anaesthetists be taught to interpret the effects of general anaesthesia on the electroencephalogram? Comparison of performance with the BIS and spectral entropy. *Br. J. Anaesth.* **2007**, *99*, 532–537. [CrossRef]
30. Chen, S.J.; Peng, C.J.; Chen, Y.C.; Hwang, Y.R.; Lai, Y.S.; Fan, S.Z.; Jen, K.K. Comparison of FFT and marginal spectra of EEG using empirical mode decomposition to monitor anesthesia. *Comput. Methods Programs Biomed.* **2016**, *137*, 77–85. [CrossRef]
31. Kreuer, S.; Wilhelm, W. The Narcotrend monitor. *Best Pract. Res. Clin. Anaesthesiol.* **2006**, *20*, 111–119. [CrossRef]
32. Kreuer, S.; Bruhn, J.; Larsen, R.; Bialas, P.; Wilhelm, W. Comparability of Narcotrend^{TM} index and bispectral index during propofol anaesthesia. *Br. J. Anaesth.* **2004**, *93*, 235–240. [CrossRef] [PubMed]
33. Kreuer, S.; Biedler, A.; Larsen, R.; Schoth, S.; Altmann, S.; Wilhelm, W. The Narcotrend—A new EEG monitor designed to measure the depth of anaesthesia. A comparison with bispectral index monitoring during propofol-remifentanil-anaesthesia. *Anaesthesist* **2001**, *50*, 921–925. [CrossRef] [PubMed]

34. Dennhardt, N.; Arndt, S.; Beck, C.; Boethig, D.; Heiderich, S.; Schultz, B.; Weber, F.; Sümpelmann, R. Effect of age on Narcotrend Index monitoring during sevoflurane anesthesia in children below 2 years of age. *Paediatr. Anaesth.* **2018**, *28*, 112–119. [CrossRef] [PubMed]
35. Dong, X.; Suo, P.; Yuan, X.; Yao, X. Use of auditory evoked potentials for intra-operative awareness in anesthesia: A consciousness-based conceptual model. *Cell Biochem. Biophys.* **2015**, *71*, 441–447. [CrossRef] [PubMed]
36. Mantzaridis, H.; Kenny, G.N. Auditory evoked potential index: A quantitative measure of changes in auditory evoked potentials during general anaesthesia. *Anaesthesia* **1997**, *52*, 1030–1036. [CrossRef]
37. Khan, J.; Mariappan, R.; Venkatraghavan, L. Entropy as an indicator of cerebral perfusion in patients with increased intracranial pressure. *J. Anaesthesiol. Clin. Pharmacol.* **2014**, *30*, 409. [CrossRef] [PubMed]
38. Illman, H.; Antila, H.; Olkkola, K.T. Reversal of neuromuscular blockade by sugammadex does not affect EEG derived indices of depth of anesthesia. *J. Clin. Monit. Comput.* **2010**, *24*, 371–376. [CrossRef]
39. Schartner, M.M.; Carhart-Harris, R.L.; Barrett, A.B.; Seth, A.K.; Muthukumaraswamy, S.D. Increased spontaneous MEG signal diversity for psychoactive doses of ketamine, LSD and psilocybin. *Sci. Rep.* **2017**, *7*, 1–12. [CrossRef] [PubMed]
40. Abdelmageed, W.M.; Al Taher, W.M. Preoperative paracetamol infusion reduces sevoflurane consumption during thyroidectomy under general anesthesia with spectral entropy monitoring. *Egypt. J. Anaesth.* **2014**, *30*, 115–122. [CrossRef]
41. Tiefenthaler, W.; Colvin, J.; Steger, B.; Pfeiffer, K.P.; Moser, P.L.; Walde, J.; Lorenz, I.H.; Kolbitsch, C. How bispectral index compares to spectral entropy of the EEG and A-line ARX index in the same patient. *Open Med.* **2018**, *13*, 583–596. [CrossRef]
42. Sullivan, C.A.; Egbuta, C.; Park, R.S.; Lukovits, K.; Cavanaugh, D.; Mason, K.P. The Use of Bispectral Index Monitoring Does Not Change Intraoperative Exposure to Volatile Anesthetics in Children. *J. Clin. Med.* **2020**, *9*, 2437. [CrossRef] [PubMed]
43. Maksimow, A.; Särkelä, M.; Långsjö, J.W.; Salmi, E.; Kaisti, K.K.; Yli-Hankala, A.; Hinkka-Yli-Salomäki, S.; Scheinin, H.; Jääskeläinen, S.K. Increase in high frequency EEG activity explains the poor performance of EEG spectral entropy monitor during S-ketamine anesthesia. *Clin. Neurophysiol.* **2006**, *117*, 1660–1668. [CrossRef]
44. Davidson, A.J.; Huang, G.H.; Rebmann, C.S.; Ellery, C. Performance of entropy and Bispectral Index as measures of anaesthesia effect in children of different ages. *Br. J. Anaesth.* **2005**, *95*, 674–679. [CrossRef] [PubMed]
45. Kim, Y.H.; Choi, W. Effect of preoperative anxiety on spectral entropy during induction with propofol. *Korean J. Anesthesiol.* **2013**, *65*, 108–113. [CrossRef] [PubMed]
46. Wu, S.; Wang, P.; Liao, W.; Shih, T.; Chang, K.; Lin, K.; Chou, A. Use of Spectral Entropy Monitoring in Reducing the Quantity of Sevoflurane as Sole Inhalational Anesthetic and in Decreasing the Need for Antihypertensive Drugs in Total Knee Replacement Surgery. *Acta Anaesthesiol. Taiwanica* **2008**, *46*, 106–111. [CrossRef]
47. Vakkuri, A.; Yli-hankala, A.; Sandin, R.; Mustola, S. Spectral Entropy Monitoring Is Associated with Reduced Propofol Use and Faster Emergence in Propofol—Nitrous Oxide—Alfentanil Anesthesia. *J. Am. Soc. Anesthesiol.* **2005**, *103*, 274–279. [CrossRef]
48. Talawar, P.; Chhabra, A.; Trikha, A.; Arora, M.K. Chandralekha Entropy monitoring decreases isoflurane concentration and recovery time in pediatric day care surgery—A randomized controlled trial. *Paediatr. Anaesth.* **2010**, *20*, 1105–1110. [CrossRef]
49. Elgebaly, A.S.; El Mourad, M.B.; Fathy, S.M. The role of entropy monitoring in reducing propofol requirements during open heart surgeries. A prospective randomized study. *Ann. Card. Anaesth.* **2020**, *23*, 272–276. [CrossRef]
50. Bhardwaj, N.; Yaddanapudi, S. A randomized trial of propofol consumption and recovery profile with BIS-guided anesthesia compared to standard practice in children. *Paediatr. Anaesth.* **2010**, *20*, 160–167. [CrossRef]
51. Aime, I.; Taylor, G. Does Monitoring Bispectral Index or Spectral Entropy Reduce Sevoflurane Use? *Anesth. Analg.* **2006**, *103*. [CrossRef]
52. Liao, W.-W.; Wang, J.-J.; Wu, G.-J.; Kuo, C.-D. The effect of cerebral monitoring on recovery after sevoflurane anesthesia in ambulatory setting in children: A comparison among bispectral index, A-line autoregressive index, and standard practice. *J. Chin. Med. Assoc.* **2011**, *74*, 28–36. [CrossRef] [PubMed]
53. Weber, F.; Geerts, N.J.E.; Roeleveld, H.G.; Warmenhoven, A.T.; Liebrand, C.A. The predictive value of the heart rate variability-derived Analgesia Nociception Index in children anaesthetized with sevoflurane: An observational pilot study. *Eur. J. Pain* **2018**, *22*, 1597–1605. [CrossRef] [PubMed]
54. Lai, R.-C.; Lu, Y.-L.; Huang, W.; Xu, M.-X.; Lai, J.-L.; Xie, J.-D.; Wang, X.-D. [Application of a narcotrend-assisted anesthesia in-depth monitor in the microwave coagulation for liver cancer during total intravenous anesthesia with propofol and fentanyl]. *Chin. J. Cancer* **2010**, *29*, 117–120. [CrossRef] [PubMed]
55. Rundshagen, I.; Hardt, T.; Cortina, K.; Pragst, F.; Fritzsche, T.; Spies, C. Narcotrend-assisted propofol/remifentanil anaesthesia vs clinical practice: Does it make a difference? *Br. J. Anaesth.* **2007**, *99*, 686–693. [CrossRef] [PubMed]
56. Sebel, P.S.; Bowdle, T.A.; Ghoneim, M.M.; Rampil, I.J.; Padilla, R.E.; Gan, T.J.; Domino, K.B. The incidence of awareness during anesthesia: A multicenter United States study. *Anesth. Analg.* **2004**, *99*, 833–839. [CrossRef]
57. Ekman, A.; Lindholm, M.-L.; Lennmarken, C.; Sandin, R. Reduction in the incidence of awareness using BIS monitoring. *Acta Anaesthesiol. Scand.* **2004**, *48*, 20–26. [CrossRef]
58. Fiedler, M.O.; Schätzle, E.; Contzen, M.; Gernoth, C.; Weiß, C.; Walter, T.; Viergutz, T.; Kalenka, A. Evaluation of Different Positive End-Expiratory Pressures Using Supreme^{TM} Airway Laryngeal Mask during Minor Surgical Procedures in Children. *Medicina* **2020**, *56*, 551. [CrossRef]

59. Bonhomme, V.; Uutela, K.; Hans, G.; Maquoi, I.; Born, J.D.; Brichant, J.F.; Lamy, M.; Hans, P. Comparison of the Surgical Pleth Index™ with haemodynamic variables to assess nociception-anti-nociception balance during general anaesthesia. *Br. J. Anaesth.* **2011**, *106*, 101–111. [CrossRef]
60. Boselli, E.; Bouvet, L.; Bégou, G.; Dabouz, R.; Davidson, J.; Deloste, J.Y.; Rahali, N.; Zadam, A.; Allaouchiche, B. Prediction of immediate postoperative pain using the analgesia/nociception index: A prospective observational study. *Br. J. Anaesth.* **2014**, *112*, 715–721. [CrossRef]
61. Ledowski, T.; Ang, B.; Schmarbeck, T.; Rhodes, J. Monitoring of sympathetic tone to assess postoperative pain: Skin conductance vs surgical stress index. *Anaesthesia* **2009**, *64*, 727–731. [CrossRef]
62. Nie, F.; Liu, T.; Zhong, L.; Yang, X.; Liu, Y.; Xia, H.; Liu, X.; Wang, X.; Liu, Z.; Zhou, L.I.; et al. MicroRNA-148b enhances proliferation and apoptosis in human renal cancer cells via directly targeting MAP3K9. *Mol. Med. Rep.* **2016**, 83–90. [CrossRef] [PubMed]
63. Jess, G.; Pogatzki-Zahn, E.M.; Zahn, P.K.; Meyer-Frießem, C.H. Monitoring heart rate variability to assess experimentally induced pain using the analgesia nociception index. *Eur. J. Anaesthesiol.* **2016**, *33*, 118–125. [CrossRef] [PubMed]
64. Edry, R.; Recea, V.; Dikust, Y.; Sessler, D.I. Preliminary Intraoperative Validation of the Nociception Level Index: A Noninvasive Nociception Monitor. *Anesthesiology* **2016**, *125*, 193–203. [CrossRef] [PubMed]
65. Gruenewald, M.; Dempfle, A. Analgesia/nociception monitoring for opioid guidance: Meta-Analysis of randomized clinical trials. *Minerva Anestesiol.* **2017**, *83*, 200–213. [CrossRef] [PubMed]
66. Wang, Y.L.; Kong, X.Q.; Ji, F.H. Effect of dexmedetomidine on intraoperative Surgical Pleth Index in patients undergoing video-assisted thoracoscopic lung lobectomy. *J. Cardiothorac. Surg.* **2020**, *15*, 1–7. [CrossRef]
67. Kim, J.H.; Jwa, E.K.; Choung, Y.; Yeon, H.J.; Kim, S.Y.; Kim, E. Comparison of Pupillometry With Surgical Pleth Index Monitoring on Perioperative Opioid Consumption and Nociception During Propofol–Remifentanil Anesthesia: A Prospective Randomized Controlled Trial. *Anesth. Analg.* **2020**, *131*, 1589–1598. [CrossRef]
68. Huiku, M.; Uutela, K.; van Gils, M.; Korhonen, I.; Kymalainen, M.; Merilainen, P.; Paloheimo, M.; Rantanen, M.; Takala, P.; Viertio-Oja, H.; et al. Assessment of surgical stress during general anaesthesia. *Br. J. Anaesth.* **2007**, *98*, 447–455. [CrossRef]
69. Dostalova, V.; Schreiberova, J.; Bartos, M.; Kukralova, L.; Dostal, P. Surgical pleth index and analgesia nociception index for intraoperative analgesia in patients undergoing neurosurgical spinal procedures: A comparative randomized study. *Minerva Anestesiol.* **2019**, *85*, 1265–1272. [CrossRef]
70. Funcke, S.; Saugel, B.; Koch, C.; Schulte, D.; Zajonz, T.; Sander, M.; Gratarola, A.; Ball, L.; Pelosi, P.; Spadaro, S.; et al. Individualized, perioperative, hemodynamic goal-directed therapy in major abdominal surgery (iPEGASUS trial): Study protocol for a randomized controlled trial. *Trials* **2018**, *19*, 273. [CrossRef]
71. Jain, N.; Gera, A.; Sharma, B.; Sood, J.; Chugh, P. Comparison of Surgical Pleth Index-guided analgesia using fentanyl versus conventional analgesia technique in laparoscopic cholecystectomy. *Minerva Anestesiol.* **2019**, *85*, 358–365. [CrossRef]
72. Won, Y.J.; Lim, B.G.; Lee, S.H.; Park, S.; Kim, H.; Lee, I.O.; Kong, M.H. Comparison of relative oxycodone consumption in surgical pleth index-guided analgesia versus conventional analgesia during sevoflurane anesthesia. *Medicina* **2016**, *95*, e4743. [CrossRef] [PubMed]
73. Chen, X.; Thee, C.; Gruenewald, M.; Ilies, C.; Höcker, J.; Hanss, R.; Steinfath, M.; Bein, B. Correlation of Surgical Pleth Index with Stress Hormones during Propofol-Remifentanil Anaesthesia. *Sci. World J.* **2012**, *2012*, 1–8. [CrossRef] [PubMed]
74. Theerth, K.A.; Sriganesh, K.; Reddy, K.M.; Chakrabarti, D.; Umamaheswara Rao, G.S. Analgesia Nociception Index-guided intraoperative fentanyl consumption and postoperative analgesia in patients receiving scalp block versus incision-site infiltration for craniotomy. *Minerva Anestesiol.* **2018**, *84*, 1361–1368. [CrossRef] [PubMed]
75. Soral, M.; Altun, G.T.; Dinçer, P.Ç.; Arslantaş, M.K.; Aykaç, Z. Effectiveness of the analgesia nociception index monitoring in patients who undergo colonoscopy with sedo-analgesia. *Turk. J. Anaesthesiol. Reanim.* **2020**, *48*, 50–57. [CrossRef] [PubMed]
76. Gall, O.; Champigneulle, B.; Schweitzer, B.; Deram, T.; Maupain, O.; Montmayeur Verchere, J.; Orliaguet, G. Postoperative pain assessment in children: A pilot study of the usefulness of the analgesia nociception index. *Br. J. Anaesth.* **2015**, *115*, 890–895. [CrossRef]
77. Jensen, E.W.; Valencia, J.F.; López, A.; Anglada, T.; Agustí, M.; Ramos, Y.; Serra, R.; Jospin, M.; Pineda, P.; Gambus, P. Monitoring hypnotic effect and nociception with two EEG-derived indices, qCON and qNOX, during general anaesthesia. *Acta Anaesthesiol. Scand.* **2014**, *58*, 933–941. [CrossRef]
78. Reich, D.L.; Hossain, S.; Krol, M.; Baez, B.; Patel, P.; Bernstein, A.; Bodian, C.A. Predictors of hypotension after induction of general anesthesia. *Anesth. Analg.* **2005**, *101*, 622–628, table of contents. [CrossRef]
79. Hug, C.C.J.; McLeskey, C.H.; Nahrwold, M.L.; Roizen, M.F.; Stanley, T.H.; Thisted, R.A.; Walawander, C.A.; White, P.F.; Apfelbaum, J.L.; Grasela, T.H. Hemodynamic effects of propofol: Data from over 25,000 patients. *Anesth. Analg.* **1993**, *77*, S21–S29.
80. Thwaites, A.; Edmends, S.; Smith, I. Inhalation induction with sevoflurane: A double-blind comparison with propofol. *Br. J. Anaesth.* **1997**, *78*, 356–361. [CrossRef]
81. Liu, T.J.; Zhang, J.C.; Gao, X.Z.; Tan, Z.B.; Wang, J.J.; Zhang, P.P.; Cheng, A.B.; Zhang, S.B. Effect of sevoflurane on the ATPase activity of hippocampal neurons in a rat model of cerebral ischemia-reperfusion injury via the cAMP-PKA signaling pathway. *Kaohsiung J. Med. Sci.* **2018**, *34*, 22–33. [CrossRef]

82. Bijker, J.B.; Van Klei, W.A.; Kappen, T.H.; Van Wolfswinkel, L.; Moons, K.G.M.; Kalkman, C.J. Incidence of intraoperative hypotension as a function of the chosen definition: Literature definitions applied to a retrospective cohort using automated data collection. *Anesthesiology* **2007**, *107*, 213–220. [CrossRef] [PubMed]
83. Chang, H.S.; Hongo, K.; Nakagawa, H. Adverse effects of limited hypotensive anesthesia on the outcome of patients with subarachnoid hemorrhage. *J. Neurosurg.* **2000**, *92*, 971–975. [CrossRef] [PubMed]
84. Monk, T.G. Processed EEG and patient outcome. *Best Pract. Res. Clin. Anaesthesiol.* **2006**, *20*, 221–228. [CrossRef] [PubMed]
85. Wesselink, E.M.; Kappen, T.H.; Torn, H.M.; Slooter, A.J.C.; van Klei, W.A. Intraoperative hypotension and the risk of postoperative adverse outcomes: A systematic review. *Br. J. Anaesth.* **2018**, *121*, 706–721. [CrossRef]
86. Ristovic, V.; de Roock, S.; Mesana, T.; van Diepen, S.; Sun, L. The Impact of Preoperative Risk on the Association between Hypotension and Mortality after Cardiac Surgery: An Observational Study. *J. Clin. Med.* **2020**, *9*, 2057. [CrossRef]
87. Walsh, M.; Kurz, A.; Turan, A.; Rodseth, R.N.; Cywinski, J.; Thabane, L.; Sessler, D.I. Relationship between Intraoperative Mean. *Anesthesiology* **2013**, *119*, 507–515. [CrossRef]
88. Bedreag, O.H.; Sandesc, D.; Chiriac, S.D.; Rogobete, A.F.; Cradigati, A.C.; Sarandan, M.; Dumache, R.; Nartita, R.; Papurica, M. The Use of Circulating miRNAs as Biomarkers for Oxidative Stress in Critically Ill Polytrauma Patients. *Clin. Lab.* **2016**, *62*, 263–274. [CrossRef]
89. Bratu, L.M.; Rogobete, A.F.; Sandesc, D.; Bedreag, O.H.; Tanasescu, S.; Nitu, R.; Popovici, S.E.; Crainiceanu, Z.P. The Use of Redox Expression and Associated Molecular Damage to Evaluate the Inflammatory Response in Critically Ill Patient with Severe Burn. *Biochem. Genet.* **2016**, *54*. [CrossRef]
90. Bedreag, O.H.; Rogobete, A.F.; Sandesc, D.; Cradigati, C.A.; Sarandan, M.; Popovici, S.E.; Dumache, R.; Horhat, F.G.; Vernic, C.; Sima, L.V.; et al. Modulation of the Redox Expression and Inflammation Response in the Critically Ill Polytrauma Patient with Thoracic Injury. Statistical Correlations between Antioxidant Therapy. *Clin. Lab.* **2016**, *62*, 1747–1759. [CrossRef]
91. Papurica, M.; Rogobete, A.F.; Sandesc, D.; Dumache, R.; Nartita, R.; Sarandan, M.; Cradigati, A.C.; Luca, L.; Vernic, C.; Bedreag, O.H. Redox Changes Induced by General Anesthesia in Critically Ill Patients with Multiple Traumas. *Mol. Biol. Int.* **2015**, *2015*, 238586. [CrossRef]
92. Dinu, A.R.; Rogobete, A.F.; Bratu, T.; Popovici, S.E.; Bedreag, O.H.; Papurica, M.; Bratu, L.M.; Sandesc, D. Cannabis Sativa Revisited—Crosstalk between microRNA Expression, Inflammation, Oxidative Stress, and Endocannabinoid Response System in Critically Ill Patients with Sepsis. *Cells* **2020**, *9*, 307. [CrossRef] [PubMed]
93. Nunes, R.R.; Nora, F.S.; Maia, D.; Dumaresq, H.; Maria, R.; Cavalcante, A.; Costa, A.A.; Moreira, L.; Carneiro, M.; Cesar, J.; et al. Influence of Total Intravenous Anesthesia, Entropy and Laparoscopy on Oxidative Stress. *Braz. J. Anesthesiol.* **2012**, *62*, 484–501. [CrossRef]
94. Gruber, J.; Fong, S.; Chen, C.; Yoong, S.; Pastorin, G.; Schaffer, S.; Cheah, I.; Halliwell, B. Mitochondria-targeted antioxidants and metabolic modulators as pharmacological interventions to slow ageing. *Biotechnol. Adv.* **2013**, *31*, 563–592. [CrossRef] [PubMed]
95. Lipina, C.; Hundal, H.S. Modulation of cellular redox homeostasis by the endocannabinoid system. *Open Biol.* **2016**, *6*, 150276. [CrossRef] [PubMed]
96. Heyland, D.K.; Dhaliwal, R.; Suchner, U.; Berger, M.M. Antioxidant nutrients: A systematic review of trace elements and vitamins in the critically ill patient. *Intensive Care Med.* **2005**, *31*, 327–337. [CrossRef]
97. Sailaja Rao, P.; Kalva, S.; Yerramilli, A.; Mamidi, S. Free Radicals and Tissue Damage: Role of Antioxidants. *Free Radic. Antioxid.* **2011**, *1*, 2–7. [CrossRef]
98. Hagar, H.H. An insight into the possible protective effect of pyrrolidine dithiocarbamate against lipopolysaccharide-induced oxidative stress and acute hepatic injury in rats. *Saudi Pharm. J.* **2009**, *17*, 259–267. [CrossRef]
99. Sorato, E.; Menazza, S.; Zulian, A.; Sabatelli, P.; Gualandi, F.; Merlini, L.; Bonaldo, P.; Canton, M.; Bernardi, P.; Di Lisa, F. Monoamine oxidase inhibition prevents mitochondrial dysfunction and apoptosis in myoblasts from patients with collagen VI myopathies. *Free Radic. Biol. Med.* **2014**, *75*, 40–47. [CrossRef]
100. Horhat, F.G.; Rogobete, A.F.; Papurica, M.; Sandesc, D.; Tanasescu, S.; Dumitrascu, V.; Licker, M.; Nitu, R.; Cradigati, C.A.; Sarandan, M.; et al. The Use of Lipid Peroxidation Expression as a Biomarker for the Molecular Damage in the Critically Ill Polytrauma Patient. *Clin. Lab.* **2016**, 1–7. [CrossRef]
101. Moise, A.; Balescu-Arion, C. The Vitamin D and the Immune System. When? Why? How? *CEACR* **2020**, *2*, 1–9. [CrossRef]
102. Georgescu, D.; Reisz, D.; Petre, I.; Ionita, I. Ischemic Stroke Secondary to Cerebral Venous Thrombosis: A Case Report. *CEACR* **2019**, 1–7. [CrossRef]
103. Timar, C.; Negrău, M.; Pantiș, C.; Daina, C.; Stanciu, S.-D.; Hodoșan, V.; Cotrău, P. Septic Shock with Chlamydia Pneumoniae Secondary to Prostatic Abscess: A Rare Case Report. *CEACR* **2019**, *1*, 1. [CrossRef]
104. Papurica, M.; Rogobete, A.F.; Sandesc, D.; Dumache, R.; Cradigati, C.A.; Sarandan, M.; Nartita, R.; Popovici, S.E.; Bedreag, O.H. Advances in biomarkers in critical ill polytrauma patients. *Clin. Lab.* **2016**, *62*, 977–986. [CrossRef]
105. Ferrari, R.S.; Andrade, C.F. Oxidative Stress and Lung Ischemia-Reperfusion Injury. *Oxidative Med. Cell. Longev.* **2015**, *2015*, 14. [CrossRef] [PubMed]
106. da Costa Paes, E.R.; Braz, M.G.; de Lima, J.T.; Gomes da Silva, M.R.; Bentes de Sousa, L.; Lima, E.S.; Carvalho de Vasconcellos, M.; Cerqueira Braz, J.R. DNA damage and antioxidant status in medical residents occupationally exposed to waste anesthetic gases. *Acta Cir. Bras.* **2014**, *29*, 280–286. [CrossRef] [PubMed]

107. Gan, T.J.; Diemunsch, P.; Habib, A.S.; Kovac, A.; Kranke, P.; Meyer, T.A.; Watcha, M.; Chung, F.; Angus, S.; Apfel, C.C.; et al. Consensus guidelines for the management of postoperative nausea and vomiting. *Anesth. Analg.* **2014**, *118*, 85–113. [CrossRef]
108. Song, D.; Hamza, M.; White, P.F.; Klein, K.; Recart, A.; Khodaparast, O. The pharmacodynamic effects of a lower-lipid emulsion of propofol: A comparison with the standard propofol emulsion. *Anesth. Analg.* **2004**, *98*, 687–691, table of contents. [CrossRef]
109. El Hor, T.; Van Der Linden, P.; De Hert, S.; Melot, C.; Bidgoli, J. Impact of entropy monitoring on volatile anesthetic uptake. *Anesthesiology* **2013**, *118*, 868–873. [CrossRef]
110. Tewari, S.; Bhadoria, P.; Wadhawan, S.; Prasad, S.; Kohli, A. Entropy vs standard clinical monitoring using total intravenous anesthesia during transvaginal oocyte retrieval in patients for in vitro fertilization. *J. Clin. Anesth.* **2016**, *34*, 105–112. [CrossRef]
111. Refaat, E.K.; Yassein, T.E. Reduced sevoflurane consumption in cirrhotic compared to non-cirrhotic patients undergoing major hepatic surgery: During entropy monitored general anesthesia. *Egypt. J. Anaesth.* **2013**, *29*, 61–65. [CrossRef]

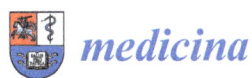

Review

Incidence of Iron Deficiency and the Role of Intravenous Iron Use in Perioperative Periods

Mirela Țiglis [1,2], **Tiberiu Paul Neagu** [3,4,*], **Andrei Niculae** [5,6], **Ioan Lascăr** [3,4] **and Ioana Marina Grințescu** [1,2]

1. Department of Anaesthesiology and Intensive Care, Emergency Clinical Hospital of Bucharest, 014461 Bucharest, Romania; mirelatiglis@gmail.com (M.Ț.); ioana.grintescu@rospen.ro (I.M.G.)
2. Clinical Department No. 14, "Carol Davila" University of Medicine and Pharmacy, 050474 Bucharest, Romania
3. Department of Plastic Surgery and Reconstructive Microsurgery, Emergency Clinical Hospital of Bucharest, 014461 Bucharest, Romania; ioan.lascar@gmail.com
4. Clinical Department No. 11, "Carol Davila" University of Medicine and Pharmacy, 050474 Bucharest, Romania
5. Department of Nephrology and Dialysis, "St. John" Emergency Clinical Hospital, 042122 Bucharest, Romania; niculaeandrei@yahoo.com
6. Clinical Department No. 3, "Carol Davila" University of Medicine and Pharmacy, 050474 Bucharest, Romania
* Correspondence: dr.neagupaul@gmail.com

Received: 26 August 2020; Accepted: 9 October 2020; Published: 12 October 2020

Abstract: Iron deficiency is a major problem in worldwide populations, being more alarming in surgical patients. In the presence of absolute iron deficiency (depletion of body iron), functional iron deficiency (during intense bone marrow stimulation by endogenous or exogenous factors), or iron sequestration (acute or chronic inflammatory conditions), iron-restricted erythropoiesis can develop. This systemic review was conducted to draw attention to the delicate problem of perioperative anemia, and to provide solutions to optimize the management of anemic surgical patients. Systemic reviews and meta-analyses, clinical studies and trials, case reports and international guidelines were studied, from a database of 50 articles. Bone marrow biopsy, serum ferritin levels, transferrin saturation, the mean corpuscular volume, and mean corpuscular hemoglobin concentration were used in the diagnosis of iron deficiency. There are various intravenous iron formulations, with different pharmacological profiles used for restoring iron. In surgical patients, anemia is an independent risk factor for morbidity and mortality. Therefore, anemia correction should be rapid, with parenteral iron formulations—the oral ones—being inefficient. Various studies showed the safety and efficacy of parenteral iron formulations in correcting hemoglobin levels and decreasing the blood transfusion rate, the overall mortality, the postoperative infections incidence, hospitalization days, and the general costs.

Keywords: iron deficiency; anemia; intravenous iron formulation; perioperative period

1. Introduction

Iron deficiency (ID), a reduction of body iron levels, is a critical problem worldwide, affecting 4–30% of men, 10–43% of all women, and reaching 52% in pregnant women. Studies showed that iron deficiency complicates the management of almost one-third of surgical patients [1]. The prevalence of preoperative anemia varies from 26 to 75%, while after major surgery, it ascends to 90% [2]. It can occur due to excessive losses in patients with massive acute bleeding or chronic hemorrhages, malabsorption, insufficient intake in relation to increased needs, or functional deficiency due to a chronic disease (e.g., HIV, cancer). In surgical patients, the cause can be multifactorial [3]. Iron deficiency might or might not be associated with anemia (a decrease in hemoglobin levels and changes in erythrocytes morphology), often being unidentified or untreated. The first phase of iron deficiency does not manifest through anemia, which usually appears in a later stage [4]. Therefore, good perioperative patient management involves monitoring hemoglobin levels and iron status before surgery and, in case of major interventions, in the postoperative period [5].

In the perioperative period, anemia is an independent factor for morbidity and mortality. It is also related to an increased incidence of red blood cell transfusion, prolonged length of stay in hospital, and higher complications [6]. Fowler et al. published a meta-analyses on the influence of preoperative anemia on patients' outcomes after major surgery, and concluded that it had a high incidence (about 39% of patients), being an independent risk factor for in-hospital mortality, acute kidney injury, and infections. In patients proposed for cardiac surgery, it was also an independent risk factor for stroke events [7].

In elective surgery, there might be enough time to correct anemia in the preoperative period, with oral and parenteral iron products or erythropoietic agents, but in major emergency surgery, there is no time for delays [6]. Anemia can also develop during hospitalization (major surgery, complications, blood sampling) and continues further after the patient's discharge, if it is not properly corrected, leading to impaired functionality on the long-term. Therefore, in order to improve patient's outcome, recent guidelines and programs promote the safety and efficacy of intravenous iron, in order to correct anemia, to reduce the need for blood transfusions, to decrease the rate of complications, and economically speaking, to reduce hospitalization costs [5,8].

2. Materials and Methods

This systemic review was conducted to draw attention to the delicate problem of perioperative anemia, to highlight the risks it has on the patients' evolution, to provide solutions for optimizing the clinical management of these surgical patients and to offer alternative solutions to blood transfusion. For this purpose, we used PUBMED database, searching for words and word combinations, in article titles or contents, like *"perioperative anemia"*, *"perioperative period"*, *"major surgery"*, *"iron deficiency"*, *"iron sequestration"*, *"intravenous iron"*, *"parenteral iron"*, *"iron molecule"*, *"iron formula"*, *"iron infusion"*, *"erythropoietic agent"*, *"blood transfusion"*, *"hypersensitivity reactions"*, and *"erythropoiesis"*. In our review, we only studied English articles, using systemic reviews and meta-analysis, clinical studies and trials, case reports, and international guidelines. A total of 50 articles (Figure 1) were included and these were reviewed by three authors (M.Ț., T.P.N., and A.N.) and two other persons (I.L., I.M.G.) checked the eligibility. The FDA network was also consulted.

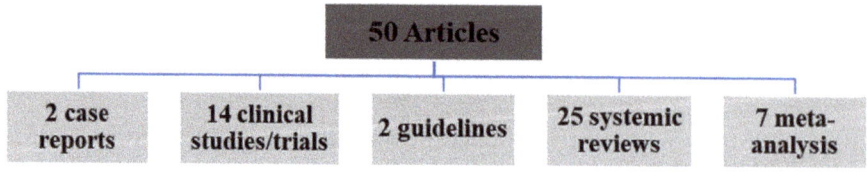

Figure 1. Articles used for analysis.

3. Results and Discussion

Parenteral iron formulations were first used in those with intolerance of, or unresponsiveness to oral iron. In the last century, intravenous iron showed its benefits in the perioperative period. It was used to rapidly correct the body iron levels and to improve hematopoiesis whenever important bleeding was anticipated or arose. Therefore, perioperative transfusion requirements and complication occurrences were reduced, improving the overall outcome of patients with chronic comorbidities [9,10].

In the following lines, important issues are presented—iron deficiency diagnosis, a short presentation of intravenous iron products, the role of parenteral iron use in the perioperative period, and the overall risks associated with intravenous iron products, in order to familiarize the clinician with the main aspects of surgical patients' anemia, acquired iron deficiency, and the existent therapeutic alternatives.

3.1. Iron Deficiency Diagnosis

Iron, a vital element, is involved in various essential biological processes of the body, like DNA synthesis, immune system functionality, erythropoiesis, hemoglobin synthesis, oxygen transport, energy metabolism, and the production of neurotransmitters [11]. Iron deficiency can commonly present as an absolute deficiency (when the iron stores are abolished) in the face of important blood loss. There can also be a functional or relative iron deficiency (increased erythropoietic response that exceeds the available iron supply) and an iron deficiency by sequestration (increased hepcidin levels, like in inflammatory diseases, induce iron retention in macrophages, or enterocytes) [12].

We should remember that iron exists in the body in many forms—circulating, stored intracellularly, and utilized, like part of the hemoglobin structure. The "gold standard" for iron deficiency diagnosis remains a bone marrow biopsy. It directly measures the iron stores that can be used in hematopoiesis, but it is a complicated, invasive, and low tolerated test that is used in rare cases. In clinical practice, the diagnosis relies mostly on serum biomarkers assessment (Table 1) [13].

Table 1. Serum biomarkers used to diagnose iron deficiency.

"Gold Standard" Method	Usual Biomarkers	Other Biomarkers
Bone marrow biopsy	Serum ferritin	Mean corpuscular volume (MCV)
	Transferrin saturation (TSAT)	Mean corpuscular haemoglobin concentration (MCHC)
	Serum iron	Red cell distribution width (RDW)
	C-reactive protein	Reticulocyte haemoglobin content (CHr)
		Zinc protoporphyrins (ZPP) in the red cell

One of the most sensitive tools for iron deficiency diagnosis is a serum ferritin level under 30 ng/mL, which is an expression of the depleted iron stores. Nevertheless, ferritin is also released when inflammation is present like in inflammatory bowel disease, autoimmune disease, or chronic renal failure, so normal, or elevated value does not always exclude iron deficiency [14,15]. Another important test is represented by transferrin saturation (TSAT), which measures the transported iron that is available for cell uptake but the reliability of TSAT in measuring iron status can also be reduced by a high inflammatory status [13]. Circulating iron, bound to its carrier (transferrin) can also be assessed, but its values can vary with the oral intake and the physiological necessities, and it can have a normal value even in the presence of depleted stores. Therefore, iron's defining parameters should be drawn after an overnight fast [14]. C-reactive protein, used to assess the patient's inflammatory status, can guide iron's deficiency diagnosis. In the presence of low ferritin (30–100 ng/mL) and transferrin saturation levels (<20%), a level of C-reactive protein below 5 mg/L is a marker of absolute iron deficiency [16].

Others markers that can be used are a low value of the mean corpuscular volume (MCV) and mean corpuscular hemoglobin concentration (MCHC) (<280 g/L). The red cell distribution width (RDW) (variation of cells volume) is increased in initial phases and after the iron treatment initiation. The reticulocyte hemoglobin content (CHr), a reflexion of iron volume available for immediate erythropoiesis, is decreased (<28 pg) [17].

3.2. Intravenous Iron Products–Short Presentation

Regarding the chemical structure, intravenous iron formulas are colloidal suspensions with a core made of iron oxyhydroxide and a stabilizer, carbohydrate shell coating. The size of the core particle influences the iron lability, the smaller size being the most labile of bound iron [18].

The various intravenous iron formulations have a similar core but the chemistry, molecular weight of the carbohydrate coat, and the bonds with the core are different. After the intravenous administration, iron molecules dissociate from the carbohydrate shell coat and binds to specific proteins. According to various studies, iron–carbohydrate complexes are taken by macrophages of the reticuloendothelial system through endocytosis. In big steps, endosome fuses with lysosome, leading to iron cleavage from the complex. Then, the iron enters the cytoplasm of the macrophages and it is incorporated into ferritin or transported out and sequestrated into transferrin. After that, iron is transported into sites of usage [19]. The new iron formulas are more stable, strongly binding the iron molecule within the carbohydrate coat, and therefore, decreasing the iron release during infusion. It allows the infusion of larger doses in comparison to older formulas (Table 2) [18,20].

Table 2. Intravenous iron formulas, usual doses, and time of administration.

Intravenous Iron Formula	Dosage and Minimum Administration Time
1. Ferric carboxymaltose (Ferinject®, Injectafer®)	1000 mg in 15 min
2. Ferric derisomaltose (Monoferric®)	1000 mg in at least 20 min (in patients > 50 kg) 20 mg/kg in at least 20 min (in patients < 50 kg)
3. Iron sucrose (Venofer®)	200 mg in 30 min
4. Low molecular weight iron dextran (LMW dextran) (Cosmofer®, InFed®)	20 mg/kg in 4–6 h
5. Sodium feeric gluconate (Ferrlecit®)	125 mg in 30–60 min
6. Ferumoxytol (Feraheme®, Rienso®)	No longer in use

Ferric derisomaltose (Monoferric®), known since 2009 as iron isomaltoside 1000 (IIM)—Monofer®, was released under this name since January 2020. It is a "new" molecule with high stability, with a carbohydrate coat made of derisomaltose, with a molecular weight of 155 kDa and a plasma half-life of approximately 27 h. The maximum dose was 20 mg/kg for patients weighing <50% and 1000 mg in patients >50 kg, with a minimum time for administration of 20 min. It could replace the total required dose in one infusion or divided doses for correcting anemia, and does not require a test dose, according to the manufacturer [3,21–23].

Ferric carboxymaltose (FCM) (Ferinject®, Injectafer®) has a carboxymaltose shell coating, with a molecular weight of 150 kDa, a high stability, and a plasma half-life of approximately 8 h. The maximum single dose is 1000 mg, administered over 15 min. It also has the ability to replace the required iron dose in a single infusion [3,24].

Iron sucrose (IS) (Venofer®) is a medium stable molecule, with a sucrose shell coating, a molecular weight of 43 kDa, a plasma half-life of 5 h, a maximum dose of 200 mg with at least 15 min minimum time for the administration. This molecule has become available for use since 2000. It needs repeated infusions to ensure the required amount of iron (about 1 g) [3,22].

Low molecular weight iron dextran (LMW dextran) (Cosmofer®, InFed®) has a dextran coat, a high stability, and 400-kDa molecular weight with a plasma half-life of about 30 h. The maximum dose is 20 mg/kg, administered over a minimum of 4–6 h. It is available in the market since 1991 [18].

Ferumoxytol (Feraheme®, Rienso®) has a polyglucose sorbitol carboxymethyl ether shell coating, with a molecular weight of 750 kDa, a high stability, and a plasma half-life of 15 h. The maximum dose is 510 mg administered over a minimum of 15 min. This product is no longer available in the European Union [18].

Sodium ferric gluconate (SFG) (Ferrlecit®), being used since 1999, is a molecule with low stability, a gluconate-made coat, a 280-kDa molecular weight, and a plasma half-life of 1 h and a half. The maximum single dose is 125 mg, with a minimum administration time of 30–60 min. It does not replace the total necessary dose, so multiple repeated infusions are required [3,18].

There is no standardized recommendations for each formula—the selection depends on availability, the prescriber's experience, the available time for correcting iron deficiency (elective or emergency surgery), the type of iron deficiency, and the patient allergenic profile [3,5,25–28].

3.3. The Role of Parenteral Iron Use in a Perioperative Period

As we previously emphasized, the perioperative period raised problems through the fact that there is no time to correct the iron deficiency with oral supplementation and many patients had zero response to these therapies due to the underlying comorbidities. Poor gastrointestinal tolerance led to the necessity of new intravenous product use in surgical patients, with a better tolerance profile, fewer adverse reactions, and rapid capacity of correcting iron deficiency [10,29,30].

A study published by Lee et al. has compared the efficacy and safety of ferric carboxymaltose (FCM) (500 mg in patients weighing <50 kg and 1000 mg in patients with >50 kg) versus iron sucrose (IS) (200 mg per session, maximum 600 mg per week), in treating preoperative anemia in gynecological patients. They concluded that 1000 mg dose of FCM leads to rapid correction of iron deficiency anemia, obtaining a hemoglobin level >10 g/dL in 7.7 days, compared to 10.5 days for IS. This allowed earlier surgical intervention, reduced the number of hospital visits (one visit for FCM, 3–8 visits for IS), and improved patient outcomes. Both formulations were safe, only being related to mild adverse events, like headaches. [31].

In cases of emergency surgery, with important bleeding or in cases requiring invasive procedures, it is recommended to restore body iron to improve postoperative recovery. High doses of parenteral iron are generally preferred (1000–1500 mg), allowing a rapid infusion (between 15 min and 1 h). For all nonselective surgical procedures, the therapy can be initiated or continued in the postoperative period [17]. Studies showed that for these cases, ferric carboxymaltose and iron isomaltoside 1000 are preferred over sodium ferric gluconate or iron sucrose. Intravenous iron administration hastened anemia correction, better replenished the iron stores, and reduced adverse event appearance, as compared to oral products [28].

In another multicenter study (IVICA trial), Keeler et al. analyzed the role of preoperative iron administration in improving the quality of life for patients after colorectal cancer surgery. Authors pointed out that the intravenous route (55 patients) is more efficient than oral iron (61 patients) in correcting hemoglobin level and improving patients' outcomes. Using the parenteral formulas, they observed rapid improvement in clinical quality of life scores on short and long-term evolution, possibly in relation to anemia correction. Intravenous iron increased the hemoglobin levels more rapidly than oral formulas, permitting an earlier surgical intervention or adjuvant therapies [32].

Intravenous iron agents have showed their usefulness in orthopedic surgery, and have become "a state of the art", as described by Muñoz et al. These are used on a daily basis in patients at risk for perioperative anemia, decreasing the need for blood transfusion and the number of transfused units, by rapidly correction the hemoglobin concentration. The postoperative recovery is hastened, the length of stay is reduced, and the cost-effectiveness is significant [33–35].

A recent meta-analysis published by Schack et al., in which 5113 studies were screened, examined the role of perioperative parenteral iron therapy in cases of acute non-cardiac surgery. A total of 3044 surgical patients (especially orthopedic interventions) were enrolled in these studies. A decrease in 30-days mortality, allogenic blood transfusion, and a lower rate of postoperative infections were observed. After the analysis, no statistical difference was observed with regards to the postoperative hemoglobin level or the hospital's length of stay [36].

3.4. The Overall Risks Associated with Intravenous Iron Products

During iron infusion, there is a risk of hypersensitivity reaction appearance or iron overload [37–39]. Studies showed that the incidence of adverse reactions is 1 in 200,000 patients, with a prevalence of <0.1% [24,40–42]. The infusion rate plays a key role. Based on experts' consensus, an infusion time extent from 15 min to one hour is recommended for the first dose. Then, the infusion time stated in the drug monograph should be respected [25].

A recent analysis, published by Achebe and DeLoughery, studied the risk of severe hypersensitivity reaction appearance related to intravenous iron used in 5247 patients. The authors concluded that there were no statistical differences regarding the severity or risk of adverse reaction appearance between various types of iron formulations [43]. Girreli et al. pointed out that if we compared the frequency and gravity of adverse events related to intravenous iron administration and red blood cell transfusion, we would observe that the rate of a major complication was lower in the iron group [3].

Mild reactions are characterized by flushing, urticaria and itching, joint pain, and chest tightness, and disappear if the infusion is stopped or the rate is lowered (Table 3) [10,44]. Cases with moderate reactions require stopping the infusion, and, in the face of marked hypotension, tachycardia, dyspnea, cough, and important chest tightness, intravenous fluids and steroids might be required [45]. Rampton et al. published a review in which they highlighted that life-threatening manifestations (cardiac arrest, wheezing, coma), which needed advanced cardiac life support, were extremely rare [46]. Delayed reactions (after 30 min since the treatment was finished) were also extremely rare. They were unspecific and manifest through fever, headache, myalgia, or arthralgia [26,47,48].

Table 3. Frequent adverse reactions related to parenteral iron administration.

Adverse Reactions	Usual Treatment
1. flushing	
2. urticaria	➢ lowering the infusion rate
3. itching	➢ stopping the infusion
4. joint pain	
5. chest tightness	

History of previous hypersensitivity reactions, atopy, and mastocytosis were cited as risk factors. There were also some elements related to increased severity of the adverse events—male sex, the concomitant use of beta-blockers or ACE inhibitors, older age and psychological liability, patients with behavioral conditions that are often non-compliant with the treatment [11,49].

A recent randomized trial, published by Wolf et al. showed that ferric carboxymaltose had a particular side effect, hypophosphatemia, being related to the stimulation of fibroblast growth factor 23 [11]. It is often asymptomatic, but in rare cases, it can lead to profound fatigue, muscle weakness, bone fractures, and osteomalacia [50,51].

4. Conclusions

The intravenous iron formulation are safe for use in the perioperative period. The use of one formula to the detriment of others is not standardized yet, the selection criteria especially being the patient profile, the prescriber's experience, the drug availability, and the time left until the surgery. The new drugs are available in a single, higher dose that allow rapid correction of anemia, granting early surgery, and reducing the number of hospital visits. The correction of iron deficiency in surgical patients is vital for overall outcome, being related with a reduced need of allogeneic blood transfusion and all associated complications, faster recovery after surgery, low rate of infections, reduced length of stay in the hospital, reduced rate of complications, and a lower cost.

Author Contributions: M.Ț., T.P.N., and A.N. contributed to data collection, analysis and interpretation, as well as to the writing of the article. I.L. and I.M.G. contributed to the critical revision. All authors have read and agreed to the published version of the manuscript.

Funding: This research received no external funding.

Conflicts of Interest: The authors declare no conflict of interest.

References

1. Pasricha, S.R.; Flecknoe-Brown, S.C.; Allen, K.J.; Gibson, P.R.; McMahon, L.P.; Olynyk, J.K.; Roger, S.D.; Savoia, H.F.; Tampi, R.; Thomson, A.R.; et al. Diagnosis and management of iron deficiency anaemia: A clinical update. *Med. J. Aust.* **2010**, *193*, 525–532. [CrossRef]
2. Munoz, M.; Acheson, A.G.; Bisbe, E.; Butcher, A.; Gómez-Ramírez, S.; Khalafallah, A.A.; Kehlet, H.; Kietaibl, S.; Liumbruno, G.M.; Meybohm, P.; et al. An international consensus statement on the management of postoperative anaemia after major surgical procedures. *Anaesthesia* **2018**, *73*, 1418–1431. [CrossRef] [PubMed]
3. Girelli, D.; Ugolini, S.; Busti, F.; Marchi, G.; Castagna, A. Modern iron replacement therapy: Clinical and pathophysiological insights. *Int. J. Hematol.* **2018**, *107*, 16–30. [CrossRef] [PubMed]
4. Longo, D.L.; Camaschella, C. Iron-deficiency anemia. *N. Engl. J. Med.* **2015**, *372*, 1832–1843. [CrossRef]
5. Elhenawy, A. Role of Preoperative Intravenous Iron Therapy to Correct Anemia before Major Surgery. *Syst. Rev.* **2018**, *4*, 29. [CrossRef] [PubMed]
6. Quinn, E.M.; Meland, E.; McGinn, S.; Anderson, J.H. Correction of iron-deficiency anaemia in colorectal surgery reduces perioperative transfusion rates: A before and after study. *Int. J. Surg.* **2017**, *38*, 1–8. [CrossRef]
7. Fowler, A.J.; Ahmad, T.; Phull, M.K.; Allard, S.; Gillies, M.A.; Pearse, R.M. Meta-analysis of the association between preoperative anaemia and mortality after surgery. *Br. J. Surg.* **2015**, *102*, 1314–1324. [CrossRef]
8. Perelman, I.; Winter, R.; Sikora, L.; Martel, G.; Saidenberg, E.; Fergusson, D. The efficacy of postoperative iron therapy in improving clinical and patient-centered outcomes following surgery: A systematic review and meta-analysis. *Transfus. Med. Rev.* **2018**, *32*, 89–101. [CrossRef]
9. Checheriță, I.A.; David, C.; Ciocâlteu, A.; Lascăr, I. Management of the chronic renal patient undergoing surgery. *Chirurgia (Bucharest, Romania: 1990)* **2009**, *104*, 525–530.
10. DeLoughery, T.G. Safety of Oral and Intravenous Iron. *Acta Haematol.* **2019**, *142*, 8–12. [CrossRef]
11. Wolf, M.; Chertow, G.M.; Macdougall, I.C.; Kaper, R.; Krop, J.; Strauss, W. Randomized trial of intravenous iron-induced hypophosphatemia. *JCI Insight* **2018**, *3*. [CrossRef] [PubMed]
12. Auerbach, M.; Goodnough, L.T.; Shander, A. Iron: The new advances in therapy. *Best Pract. Res. Clin. Anaesthesiol.* **2013**, *27*, 131–140. [CrossRef] [PubMed]
13. Kang, C.K.; Pope, M.; Lang, C.C.; Kalra, P.R. Iron deficiency in heart failure: Efficacy and safety of intravenous iron therapy. *Cardiovasc. Ther.* **2017**, *35*, e12301. [CrossRef] [PubMed]
14. Goodnough, L.T.; Nemeth, E.; Ganz, T. Detection, evaluation, and management of iron-restricted erythropoiesis. *Blood* **2010**, *116*, 4754–4761. [CrossRef] [PubMed]
15. Niculae, A.; David, C.; Dragomirescu, R.F.; Peride, I.; Turcu, F.L.; Petcu, L.C.; Covic, A.; Checherita, I.A. Correlation between recombinant human erythropoietin dose and inflammatory status in dialysed patients. *Rev. Chim. Buchar.* **2017**, *68*, 354–357. [CrossRef]
16. Gómez-Ramírez, S.; Bisbe, E.; Shander, A.; Spahn, D.R.; Muñoz, M. Management of Perioperative Iron Deficiency Anemia. *Acta Haematol.* **2019**, *142*, 21–29. [CrossRef]
17. Camaschella, C. Iron deficiency: New insights into diagnosis and treatment. *Hematology* **2015**, *2015*, 8–13. [CrossRef]
18. Gupta, A.; Pratt, R.D.; Crumbliss, A.L. Ferrous iron content of intravenous iron formulations. *Biometals* **2016**, *29*, 411–415. [CrossRef]
19. Worm, M.; Francuzik, W.; Renaudin, J.M.; Bilo, M.B.; Cardona, V.; Scherer Hofmeier, K.; Köhli, A.; Bauer, A.; Christoff, G.; Cichocka-Jarosz, E.; et al. Factors increasing the risk for a severe reaction in anaphylaxis: An analysis of data from The European Anaphylaxis Registry. *Allergy* **2018**, *73*, 1322–1330. [CrossRef]
20. Auerbach, M.; Macdougall, I. The available intravenous iron formulations: History, efficacy, and toxicology. *Hemodial. Int.* **2017**, *21*, S83–S92. [CrossRef]

21. Kei, T.; Mistry, N.; Curley, G.; Pavenski, K.; Shehata, N.; Tanzini, R.M.; Gauthier, M.F.; Thorpe, K.; Schweizer, T.A.; Ward, S.; et al. Efficacy and safety of erythropoietin and iron therapy to reduce red blood cell transfusion in surgical patients: A systematic review and meta-analysis. *Can. J. Anesth./J. Can. D'anesth.* **2019**, *66*, 716–731. [CrossRef] [PubMed]
22. Martin-Malo, A.; Borchard, G.; Flühmann, B.; Mori, C.; Silverberg, D.; Jankowska, E.A. Differences between intravenous iron products: Focus on treatment of iron deficiency in chronic heart failure patients. *ESC Heart Fail.* **2019**, *6*, 241–253. [CrossRef]
23. Available online: https://www.accessdata.fda.gov/drugsatfda_docs/label/2020/208171s000lbl.pdf (accessed on 21 September 2020).
24. Neiser, S.; Rentsch, D.; Dippon, U.; Kappler, A.; Weidler, P.G.; Göttlicher, J.; Steininger, R.; Wilhelm, M.; Braitsch, M.; Funk, F.; et al. Physico-chemical properties of the new generation IV iron preparations ferumoxytol, iron isomaltoside 1000 and ferric carboxymaltose. *Biometals* **2015**, *28*, 615–635. [CrossRef] [PubMed]
25. Larson, D.S.; Coyne, D.W. Update on intravenous iron choices. *Curr. Opin. Nephrol. Hypertens.* **2014**, *23*, 186–191. [CrossRef] [PubMed]
26. Lim, W.; Afif, W.; Knowles, S.; Lim, G.; Lin, Y.; Mothersill, C.; Nistor, I.; Rehman, F.; Song, C.; Xenodemetropoulos, T. Canadian expert consensus: Management of hypersensitivity reactions to intravenous iron in adults. *Vox Sang.* **2019**, *114*, 363–373. [CrossRef]
27. Szebeni, J.; Fishbane, S.; Hedenus, M.; Howaldt, S.; Locatelli, F.; Patni, S.; Rampton, D.; Weiss, G.; Folkersen, J. Hypersensitivity to intravenous iron: Classification, terminology, mechanisms and management. *British J. Pharmacol.* **2015**, *172*, 5025–5036. [CrossRef]
28. Muñoz, M.; Gómez-Ramírez, S.; Bhandari, S. The safety of available treatment options for iron-deficiency anemia. *Expert Opin. Drug Saf.* **2018**, *17*, 149–159. [CrossRef]
29. Keating, G.M. Ferric carboxymaltose: A review of its use in iron deficiency. *Drugs* **2015**, *75*, 101–127. [CrossRef]
30. Casteleyn, I.; Joosten, E. Evaluation of Parenteral Iron Therapy in Ambulatory Older Adults with Iron Deficiency Anaemia. *Acta Haematol.* **2017**, *138*, 221–222. [CrossRef]
31. Lee, S.; Ryu, K.J.; Lee, E.S.; Lee, K.H.; Lee, J.J.; Kim, T. Comparative efficacy and safety of intravenous ferric carboxymaltose and iron sucrose for the treatment of preoperative anemia in patients with menorrhagia: An open-label, multicenter, randomized study. *J. Obstet. Gynaecol. Res.* **2019**, *45*, 858–864. [CrossRef]
32. Keeler, B.D.; Dickson, E.A.; Simpson, J.A.; Ng, O.; Padmanabhan, H.; Brookes, M.J.; Acheson, A.G.; IVICA Trial Group; Banerjea, A.; Walter, C.; et al. The impact of pre-operative intravenous iron on quality of life after colorectal cancer surgery: Outcomes from the intravenous iron in colorectal cancer-associated anaemia (IVICA) trial. *Anaesthesia* **2019**, *74*, 714–725. [CrossRef] [PubMed]
33. Gómez-Ramírez, S.; Maldonado-Ruiz, M.Á.; Campos-Garrigues, A.; Herrera, A.; Muñoz, M. Short-term perioperative iron in major orthopedic surgery: State of the art. *Vox Sang.* **2019**, *114*, 3–16. [CrossRef] [PubMed]
34. Muñoz, M.; Breymann, C.; García-Erce, J.A.; Gómez-Ramírez, S.; Comin, J.; Bisbe, E. Efficacy and safety of intravenous iron therapy as an alternative/adjunct to allogeneic blood transfusion. *Vox Sang.* **2008**, *94*, 172–183. [CrossRef] [PubMed]
35. Parker, M.J. Iron supplementation for anemia after hip fracture surgery: A randomized trial of 300 patients. *JBJS* **2010**, *92*, 265–269. [CrossRef]
36. Schack, A.; Berkfors, A.A.; Ekeloef, S.; Gögenur, I.; Burcharth, J. The Effect of Perioperative Iron Therapy in Acute Major Non-cardiac Surgery on Allogenic Blood Transfusion and Postoperative Haemoglobin Levels: A Systematic Review and Meta-analysis. *World J. Surg.* **2019**, *43*, 1677–1691. [CrossRef]
37. Schrier, S.L.; Bacon, B.R. *Approach to the Patient with Suspected Iron Overload*; Official Topic from UpToDate; UpToDate: Waltham, MA, USA, 2016.
38. Çinarsoy, M.; Günes, A.K.; Gözden, H.E. ACUTE IRON OVERLOAD WITH IRON CARBOXYMALTOSE: CASE REPORT: PB2048. *Hemasphere* **2019**, *3*, 924. [CrossRef]
39. Ramanathan, G.; Olynyk, J.K.; Ferrari, P. Diagnosing and preventing iron overload. *Hemodial. Int.* **2017**, *21*, S58–S67. [CrossRef]
40. Bircher, A.J.; Auerbach, M. Hypersensitivity from intravenous iron products. *Immunol. Allergy Clin.* **2014**, *34*, 707–723. [CrossRef]

41. Muñoz, M.; Gómez-Ramírez, S.; García-Erce, J.A. Intravenous iron in inflammatory bowel disease. *World J. Gastroenterol. WJG* **2009**, *15*, 4666. [CrossRef]
42. Silverstein, S.B.; Rodgers, G.M. Parenteral iron therapy options. *Am. J. Hematol.* **2004**, *76*, 74–78. [CrossRef]
43. Achebe, M.; DeLoughery, T.G. Clinical data for intravenous iron–debunking the hype around hypersensitivity. *Transfusion* **2020**. [CrossRef] [PubMed]
44. Auerbach, M.; Deloughery, T. Single-dose intravenous iron for iron deficiency: A new paradigm. *Hematology* **2016**, *1*, 57–66. [CrossRef] [PubMed]
45. Vaucher, P.; Druais, P.L.; Waldvogel, S.; Favrat, B. Effect of iron supplementation on fatigue in nonanemic menstruating women with low ferritin: A randomized controlled trial. *Cmaj* **2012**, *184*, 1247–1254. [CrossRef] [PubMed]
46. Rampton, D.; Folkersen, J.; Fishbane, S.; Hedenus, M.; Howaldt, S.; Locatelli, F.; Patni, S.; Szebeni, J.; Weiss, G. Hypersensitivity reactions to intravenous iron: Guidance for risk minimization and management. *Haematologica* **2014**, *99*, 1671–1676. [CrossRef] [PubMed]
47. Lee, A.Y.; Leung, S.H. Safety profile of iron polymaltose infusions. *Hosp. Pract.* **2019**, *47*, 96–98. [CrossRef]
48. Qunibi, W.Y. The efficacy and safety of current intravenous iron preparations for the management of iron-deficiency anaemia: A review. *Arzneimittelforschung* **2010**, *60*, 399–412. [CrossRef]
49. Negoescu, I.; Niculescu, D.A.; David, C.; Peride, I.; Niculae, A.; Checherita, I.A.; Poiana, C. Biochemical determinants of aggressive behaviour–patho-physiological connections in esrdand dialysis. *Farmacia* **2018**, *66*, 925–929. [CrossRef]
50. Anand, G.; Schmid, C. Severe hypophosphataemia after intravenous iron administration. *Case Rep.* **2017**, *2017*, bcr2016219160. [CrossRef]
51. Zoller, H.; Schaefer, B.; Glodny, B. Iron-induced hypophosphatemia: An emerging complication. *Curr. Opin. Nephrol. Hypertens.* **2017**, *26*, 266–275. [CrossRef]

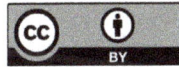

© 2020 by the authors. Licensee MDPI, Basel, Switzerland. This article is an open access article distributed under the terms and conditions of the Creative Commons Attribution (CC BY) license (http://creativecommons.org/licenses/by/4.0/).

MDPI
St. Alban-Anlage 66
4052 Basel
Switzerland
Tel. +41 61 683 77 34
Fax +41 61 302 89 18
www.mdpi.com

Medicina Editorial Office
E-mail: medicina@mdpi.com
www.mdpi.com/journal/medicina

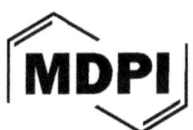

www.ingramcontent.com/pod-product-compliance
Lightning Source LLC
LaVergne TN
LVHW070541100526
838202LV00012B/343